Screening in primary health care

Screening in primary health care

Setting priorities with limited resources

Paula A. Braveman
Family and Community Medicine
University of California,
San Francisco, CA, USA

&

E. Tarimo
Division of Strengthening of Health Services
World Health Organization,
Geneva, Switzerland

World Health Organization
Geneva
1994

WHO Library Cataloguing in Publication Data

Braveman, Paula A.
  Screening in primary health care : setting priorities with limited
  resources / Paula A. Braveman & E. Tarimo.

  1.Health status 2.Diagnosis 3.Health priorities 4.Primary prevention 5.Primary health care I.Tarimo,
  E. II.Title

  ISBN 92 4 154473 2   (NLM Classification: WB 141.4)

The World Health Organization welcomes requests for permission to reproduce or translate its publications, in part or in full. Applications and enquiries should be addressed to the Office of Publications, World Health Organization, Geneva, Switzerland, which will be glad to provide the latest information on any changes made to the text, plans for new editions, and reprints and translations already available.

The designations employed and the presentation of the material in this publication do not imply the expression of any opinion whatsoever on the part of the Secretariat of the World Health Organization concerning the legal status of any country, territory, city or area or of its authorities, or concerning the delimitation of its frontiers or boundaries.

The mention of specific companies or of certain manufacturers' products does not imply that they are endorsed or recommended by the World Health Organization in preference to others of a similar nature that are not mentioned. Errors and omissions excepted, the names of proprietary products are distinguished by initial capital letters.

The authors alone are responsible for the views expressed in this publication.

TYPESET IN INDIA
PRINTED IN ENGLAND
93/9812–Macmillan/Clays–6500

Contents

Foreword

Health promotion and disease prevention are increasingly viewed as essential for improving the health of populations. Several approaches exist for delivering preventive services and promoting healthy lifestyles. One is centred on the patient/physician interaction and uses the clinical encounter to promote primary and secondary preventive services. This approach, although important, needs to be complemented by population and community-based efforts.

My interest in the subject of this book goes back to my participation in the Canadian Task Force on the Periodic Health Examination. This Task Force was created in the late 1970s in Canada with the specific mandate of examining the world literature on clinical prevention and formulating specific recommendations to health care practitioners and their patients on the use of preventive interventions. The Task Force developed a methodology for examining the efficacy and effectiveness of preventive interventions based on studies done in the field. In 1984, the US Preventive Services Task Force was created with a similar mandate and the two Task Forces established a productive and fruitful collaboration, sharing methodologies and in several instances issuing similar recommendations.

Clearly, many aspects of recommendations developed and issued in North America may not be applicable to other countries, particularly developing countries. The health situation in developing countries is quite different from that in industrialized countries, as witnessed by disparities in health indicators and health care spending around the world. In addition, many developing countries are in the midst of an epidemiological transition and hence have to tackle infectious diseases as well as the emerging threat of chronic diseases such as cardiovascular diseases and cancer. Any attempt to formulate recommendations for preventive services in developing countries has to be nested in the social and health situation of these countries. The task is huge and complex.

This publication is an initial attempt to look at preventive services in the light of the situation in developing countries, and to examine their efficacy and effectiveness using a method that considers scientific evidence as well as crucial programme and policy issues. The authors have undertaken an extensive review of available literature, including unpublished material of the World Health Organization, and conducted a critical reassessment of general issues pertaining to preventive services from the perspective of the needs of decision-makers in developing countries. They have amassed and organized a wide range of material, examining it from a fresh perspective and with an understanding of important global concerns. They have called into question many assumptions that have been insufficiently examined before and have suggested a useful framework within which specific issues can be approached in particular settings.

The authors have made an admirable attempt at a difficult task. Their effort should be commended and viewed as the beginning of an exciting itinerary that should lead to a critical examination of preventive services in developing countries. Indeed, the ideas and approaches explored here need to be developed further, tested thoroughly under particular conditions, and translated into specific recommendations that fit specific circumstances.

This publication does not claim to be the definitive word on prevention in developing countries but is an important contribution to an extensive process that should unfold at different levels. It should be viewed as a working document for those interested in going forward and further in the assessment of the efficacy and effectiveness of preventive interventions, clinical and community-based, as they apply to developing countries. It could be used as a reference document by any group operating at an international, national, regional, or local level whose purpose would be to try to delineate those interventions that could be implemented.

Whereas science and policy making are very different endeavours, any attempt to enhance the links between them should be applauded. This book is a good example of technology assessment applied to the area of prevention and for developing countries. It is a flagship for more initiatives of this sort to emerge not only in the area of preventive services but also for other clinical and community health interventions.

Renaldo N. Battista
Director, Division of Clinical Epidemiology
The Montreal General Hospital, McGill University
Montreal, Quebec, Canada

Acknowledgements

Key advisers

The authors are particularly grateful to the following persons, not only for reviewing draft material in detail and suggesting revisions, but also for contributing ideas which have had a significant influence on the development of this publication.

Renaldo Battista, Vice Chairman, Canadian Task Force on the Periodic Health Examination, and Associate Professor, McGill University, Montreal, Canada;

John Shao, Professor and Chair, Department of Microbiology and Immunology, Muhimbili Medical Centre, Dar Es Salaam, United Republic of Tanzania

Barbara Starfield, Professor and Head, Division of Health Policy, Johns Hopkins University School of Public Health, Baltimore, MD, USA.

Within the World Health Organization, Dr Jan Stjernswärd and Dr Ivan Gyárfás of the Division of Noncommunicable Diseases made especially important contributions; their work and that of colleagues in their Division helped to frame the conceptual basis for this project.

Additional assistance

In addition to the above-mentioned key advisers, the authors also thank the following for their detailed criticisms and conceptual guidance, and for making available their own and colleagues' work. The institutions mentioned are those to which these persons were attached at the time they assisted us with this undertaking.

Dr L. Arguello, School of Public Health of Nicaragua, Managua, Nicaragua
Dr M. Belsey, Family Health, WHO, Geneva, Switzerland
Mr A. Creese, Strengthening of Health Services, WHO, Geneva, Switzerland
Dr D. Egger, Strengthening of Health Services, WHO, Geneva, Switzerland
Mr S. Fluss, Health Legislation, WHO, Geneva, Switzerland
Dr R. Guidotti, Family Health, WHO, Geneva, Switzerland
Dr T. Gyorkos, McGill University, Montreal, Canada
Dr T. Hall, University of California, San Francisco, CA, USA
Dr J. Heikel, Faculty of Medicine of Casablanca, Morocco, and McGill University, Montreal, Canada

Dr A. Issakov, Strengthening of Health Services, WHO, Geneva, Switzerland

Dr H. Kahssay, Strengthening of Health Services, WHO, Geneva, Switzerland

Mrs M.-H. LeClercq, Oral Health, WHO, Geneva, Switzerland

Dr E. Liisberg, Health and Biomedical Information, WHO, Geneva, Switzerland

Dr J. Martin, Strengthening of Health Services, WHO, Geneva, Switzerland

Dr E. Najera, Pan American Health Organization/World Health Organization, Buenos Aires, Argentina

Dr M.I. Roemer, University of California, Los Angeles, CA, USA

Dr P.M. Shah, Family Health, WHO, Geneva, Switzerland

Dr I. Tabibzadeh, Strengthening of Health Services, WHO, Geneva, Switzerland

Dr S. Woolf, Scientific Adviser to the US Preventive Services Task Force, Washington, DC, USA

In addition, we wish to thank the following persons who provided assistance in identifying reference material:

Dr T. Bennett, University of California, San Francisco, CA, USA

Dr T. Imai, Director-General's Office, WHO, Geneva, Switzerland

Dr D. Kamerow, US Preventive Services Task Force, Washington, DC, USA

Dr C. Montoya, Strengthening of Health Services, WHO, Geneva, Switzerland

Dr O. P. Shchepin, Institute for Research on Social Hygiene, Public Health Economics and Management, Moscow, Russian Federation

Dr A.E. Washington, University of California, San Francisco, CA, USA

Mr T. Webster, Strengthening of Health Services, WHO, Geneva, Switzerland

Ms K. Marchi, University of California, San Francisco, CA, USA provided assistance with editing.

We are also grateful to the following persons who assisted in locating references, in arranging meetings and communications, and in preparing this publication:

Mrs C. Allaman, Strengthening of Health Services, WHO, Geneva, Switzerland

Mr R. Lynch, University of California, San Francisco, CA, USA

Mrs A. Pollinger, Strengthening of Health Services, WHO, Geneva, Switzerland

Mr W. Tsang, University of California, San Francisco, CA, USA

The financial support of the Danish International Development Agency is gratefully acknowledged.

Introduction

The purpose of this publication

Early detection practices have become a routine component of health services in every country in the world. One such practice, health screening, is designed to seek out people likely to have a health problem but who are asymptomatic and thus would not seek care for the problem at that particular time. The goal of screening is to intervene in a timely manner to deal with any inapparent risks or diseases detected, subject to confirmation by other detection methods if the screening procedure is not diagnostic in itself. Health care policy-makers in developing as well as industrialized countries are now frequently faced with decisions on whether, when, or how to introduce screening activities into routine health services.

Recent publications (USPSTF, 1989; CTF, 1979, 1984, 1986, 1989, 1990, 1991) have summarized the conclusions reached in comprehensive, systematic, and intensive reviews of evidence on the potential benefits and risks of many routine procedures used to screen persons for health problems in highly industrialized countries, thus providing guidance for policy-makers and clinicians in such countries. However, there is no recent literature dealing with the general subject of health screening in the developing countries. In the absence of relevant alternative sources, policy-makers in developing countries are often under pressure to adopt recommendations put forward by the available sources that appear most authoritative scientifically. Such pressure operates despite misgivings about the relevance of the available references to prevailing local conditions.

Expensive modalities of medical care employing high technology have proliferated in industrialized countries in recent decades; such technology has an inevitable lure for developing nations as well. The "health transition" is a term used to denote the shift in the morbidity and mortality profile of a developing nation from one overwhelmingly dominated by acute infectious diseases and short life expectancy towards one in which there is an increasing burden of chronic noncommunicable disease in an aging, more urbanized population. This phenomenon has compounded the dilemmas facing health policy-makers in developing countries when deciding on investment in technology. On the one hand, with the health transition, pressure has become increasingly strong to adopt approaches used in industrialized countries, including high technology procedures for the early detection of cancer and other noncommunicable diseases. Such pressure tends to come from those population groups, generally urban and relatively privileged, that use clinical

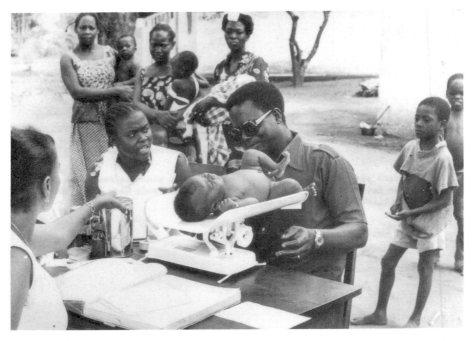

Screening for infant growth in a well-baby programme.   (WHO/18212)

services most and understandably want the highest quality of care. At the same time, however, in the course of the health transition, the overall resources of developing countries have generally increased minimally, if at all. Furthermore, the burden of infectious disease and many forms of suffering whose causes are preventable by measures that use relatively low technology remains distressingly high in developing countries, especially in rural areas and among urban slum dwellers. The diversion of limited resources towards modalities employing higher technology may thus prove detrimental to the most vulnerable sectors of the population.

This publication is an attempt to place health screening within the context of the principles of primary health care, a strategy discussed in Chapter 1. The primary health care strategy prioritizes the use of technology and all available resources in the most equitable, efficient, and effective way. The goal of this publication is to increase the likelihood of screening being used as a tool within that strategy and of its not being used when other methods would be more productive.

We see this effort as a beginning, not as an end-point. The intention is not to provide definitive answers but to raise important questions and recommend an approach to decision-making that can be applied by policy-makers and programme managers to their own specific circumstances. While it is hoped that this publication will be of interest to clinicians, it is not intended to serve as

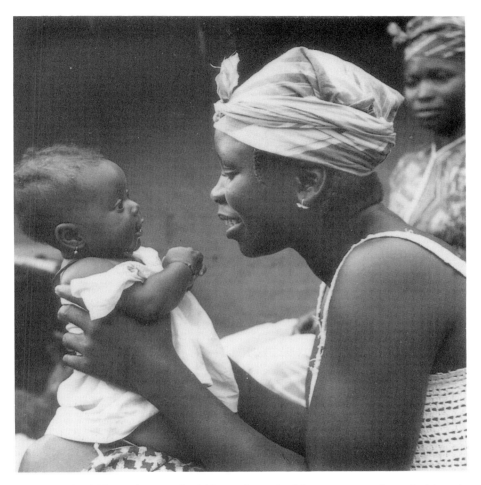

Screening should be used as a tool within a primary health care strategy that prioritizes the use of resources in the most equitable, efficient, and effective way. (WHO/18430)

a guide to clinical practice. Guidelines on practice must be developed at the appropriate level within each country, taking account of local conditions and needs. If this publication serves its purpose, it will raise questions and stimulate interest, thus helping to initiate a process leading to the development and continuing reassessment of policies and guidelines on practice in many settings. Although the book is mainly addressed to decision-makers in developing countries, we believe that the primary health care strategy has much to offer policy-makers in industrialized countries as well. This is true whenever inequities and problems associated with poverty exist, and is especially so where there is no national health care programme guaranteeing access to basic preventive and curative services for the entire population, regardless of ability to pay.

Comparison with other works assessing health screening

This publication is distinct from previous work on health screening in scope, methods, and objectives. It was not within the scope of our project to evaluate the scientific quality of the studies used as references. The stated recommendations on screening were developed, after a review of the literature and consultation with experts, to illustrate the application of a recommended approach rather than as definitive prescriptions. In contrast, national task forces in Canada (the Canadian Task Force on the Periodic Health Examination) and the USA (the US Preventive Services Task Force) set up large consensus panels which systematically assessed the quality of the evidence, using the assessments as a basis for clinical practice recommendations on a range of preventive services, including screening, in the North American setting. A similar task on a somewhat smaller scale was recently undertaken by a large working party which assessed the health screening of children in the United Kingdom (Butler, 1989; Hall, 1989). A book published by the Nuffield Trust (Holland & Stewart, 1990) takes a thoughtful look at screening for all age groups within the context of health services in the United Kingdom and has considerable relevance for other industrialized countries with national health programmes. Although no large task forces took part in its preparation, its authors provide an intensive review of the quality of the scientific evidence for and against the use of particular screening tests.

The present work differs from most of the earlier efforts in the field in that it is explicitly aimed at policy-makers rather than clinicians; it is also unique among such efforts in that it is primarily concerned with the needs of developing countries. This has led to an emphasis on the wider economic and social implications of any decision to incorporate a given early detection activity directed at asymptomatic individuals into routine health services. Particular attention has been paid to questions of access, equity, and long-term social and economic development, along with the technical and ethical issues addressed in earlier literature.

This publication is divided into eight chapters.

- Chapter 1 discusses how health screening has been viewed to date, briefly explains primary health care, and poses the crucial questions that arise when screening is assessed from the standpoint of primary health care.
- In Chapter 2, we recommend a series of criteria to guide decision-making on whether or not to use health screening as part of an approach to the prevention of a given health problem.
- Chapter 3 presents principles to be applied in the planning and implementation of health services using screening, once it has been decided that the use of screening would be advisable.
- Chapters 5 through 8 review selected examples of the potential use of screening in relation to the concerns and criteria presented in the previous chapters, in order to illustrate the application of the recommended approach and to suggest options for consideration. For each of the screening practices reviewed, there is a recommendation on whether

priority should be given to its possible adoption as part of a primary health care approach to prevention. The recommendations are intended to generate discussion and new research, and are not definitive prescriptions. The methodology used to arrive at them is discussed in Chapter 4. Summary tables are presented after the review of screening practices (pp. 139–164).

CHAPTER 1

Reassessing health screening from a primary health care standpoint

Definition and scope of health screening

> Health screening: Presumptive methods for actively seeking to identify unrecognized health risks or asymptomatic disease for timely intervention.

Health screening can be defined as the use of presumptive methods to identify unrecognized health risk factors or asymptomatic disease in persons determined by prior studies to be potentially at elevated risk and able to benefit from interventions performed before overt symptoms develop. Screening is usually more rapid and less costly than definitive diagnosis, and positive screening results often require confirmatory diagnostic tests. The subject of this publication is prescriptive screening, i.e., screening performed in order to

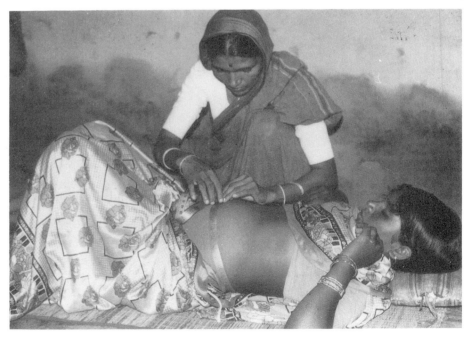

Screening techniques include enquiry, observation, and physical examination with and without the use of instruments, as well as laboratory methods.   (A. Pratinidhi/WHO/19597)

direct preventive or curative activities to those who are screened and can benefit from timely interventions that are feasible under local conditions. Unless otherwise specified, it should be assumed that when the term "screening" is used, it refers to prescriptive screening. The term "health screening" and other terms and abbreviations frequently used in this publication are defined in the Glossary (page 165).

A screening activity should never be thought of as a service in itself. Screening is a component of a wider strategy which may include definitive diagnosis and always includes a plan of action for health promotion and the prevention or control of disease. For example, screening for cervical cancer is useless unless resources are in place to provide effective follow-up and treatment for those found to have cancerous or precancerous lesions. At times we refer to a screening-diagnosis-and-timely-intervention or, for brevity, a screening-and-timely-intervention strategy. Any screening procedure needs to be thought of as part of a sequence of activities culminating in effective action at the primary, secondary, or tertiary levels of prevention. Prevention and its levels are discussed later in this chapter and defined in the Glossary (page 167).

Early detection is a broader term encompassing screening, case-finding (detecting disease in a person presenting for care for other reasons) and other approaches to early detection, such as mass campaigns to educate the public to consult the available clinical services when easily recognizable signs or symptoms occur. The line between symptomatic and asymptomatic may be blurred at times, however. In settings where access is extremely limited, many signs or symptoms, even quite serious and painful ones, may be considered normal because services for their treatment or prevention have not historically been accessible and the population has thus come to see them as an inevitable part of life. Blindness due to onchocerciasis in endemic areas is a striking example, as is gross haematuria due to bladder infection with schistosomes in regions where schistosomiasis is endemic, or even grotesquely large goitres in areas of endemic iodine deficiency. Even in industrialized countries, among population groups with low income and a low level of education, and with limited access to health care, many older people needlessly suffer blindness due to cataracts, and postmenopausal women endure urinary incontinence due to uterine prolapse. This occurs because of a belief among those affected or those caring for them that the symptoms are normal for people of that age and not indicative of disease.

In this publication, therefore, we have occasionally construed screening very broadly to include any practice for presumptive early detection of health problems that are not apparent to the individuals concerned. This may include early detection of diseases with symptoms that people with greater health knowledge and access to care would have identified as pathological. Strictly speaking, however, such practices fall into the category of early detection rather than that of screening, which should refer only to detection of asymptomatic conditions. Generally, where health problems have characteristic symptoms that would be easily recognizable in an informed population, we recommend using public education to promote self-referral to easily accessible medical care services as the appropriate strategy for secondary prevention, rather than depending on screening as strictly defined. However, when we explicitly contrast health screening with early detection, it should be understood that we are making a distinction between the screening of asymptomatic persons and the early detection of symptomatic conditions.

The term "screening" often suggests the use of laboratory tests to detect specific diseases or their precursors. It can, however, be used, as we have used it here, to refer to the application of a wide range of methods for the presumptive identification of diverse risks to health status. Screening techniques include enquiry, observation, and physical examination with and without the use of instruments, as well as laboratory methods; in this publication, a "test" means any type of detection procedure.

Screening activities can also be carried out for research purposes. The information gained may be helpful in population monitoring and programme planning, i.e., for reassessing existing priorities and setting new ones. But prescriptive screening has a purpose distinct from that of epidemiological studies describing the incidence, prevalence or natural history of a disease in a population. Indeed, the effective use of health screening depends on the existence of prior epidemiological knowledge of the natural history of, and major risk factors for, disease in the general population, as well as on knowledge of the distribution of important risk factors (socioeconomic, environmental) in local populations. This prior knowledge is needed to identify the groups likely to be at greatest risk who should be given priority to receive screening and appropriate follow-up (i.e., definitive diagnosis and effective intervention). In Chapter 3, we discuss the targeting of services involving screening, including preliminary risk assessment at the community level.

Since many health risks are shared by members of a household or a community, screening persons at the household or community level (e.g., in neighbourhoods or workplaces) is often an effective approach. Furthermore, regardless of whether it is conducted at the individual level in health facilities or in a household or community setting, screening may detect risks that require preventive action at the individual, household, or community level. Many risks detected in individuals by health care providers reveal problems at the family or community level, for example, the malnourished child whose condition points to a family (perhaps including other children or a pregnant woman) with an unemployed head of household or to poor food supply in an entire community. A population-based approach to screening should assist providers of health care to determine the most appropriate level or levels at which timely action should be taken.

Routine environmental surveillance is an important form of early detection involving assessment of environmental conditions in order to detect potential causes of adverse health effects before damage has occurred. Examples include workplace, marketplace, or neighbourhood surveillance for inapparent health hazards and routine monitoring of drinking-water, waste disposal, and housing conditions. Continuous surveillance of inapparent environmental hazards with timely intervention to prevent hazardous exposure of individuals, families, and

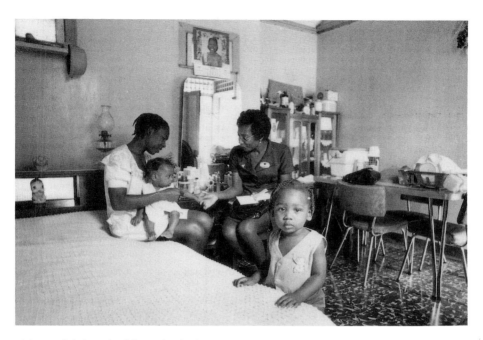

A home visit by a health worker in Jamaica. Home visiting permits a broad assessment of risks to health at the household level, as well as the delivery of other preventive services such as education and support. (J. Littlewood/WHO/16788)

communities is essential for health promotion and disease prevention. A detailed consideration of environmental surveillance is beyond the scope of this publication, but it should be seen as complementary to health screening.

Responding to the risks found on screening

Effective preventive action may or may not involve health services (see box, page 10). Health workers tend to think of early detection techniques as being used to detect diseases or associated risk factors that the health sector is equipped to address effectively. But health screening may detect health problems requiring action that is beyond the scope of the health sector. Examples include: widespread malnutrition in a community due to inadequate food supply; recurrent infant diarrhoea associated with inadequate water supply and unhygienic conditions; or high rates of schistosomal infection of the urinary tract from exposure to snail-infested water. Intervention through the health services alone will have little or no lasting effect. In such cases, the involvement of the community itself is essential to finding effective ways of dealing with the problems detected.

Prevention

Prevention is generally thought of as occurring at three possible levels: primary, secondary, and tertiary.

- Primary prevention means limiting the occurrence of a health problem, generally by preventing exposure to known risk factors. Examples include: preventing schistosomiasis by preventing people from coming into contact with water infested with snails; reducing levels of malnutrition through social and economic reforms to increase access to adequate food; or preventing lung cancer through legislation and education to discourage young people from starting to smoke.
- Secondary prevention involves action to limit the adverse consequences of disease by intervening before symptoms have occurred or during their early stages. Secondary prevention thus involves early detection (and possibly screening, if individuals are asymptomatic) and curative action. Examples include: preventing invasive carcinoma of the uterine cervix by detecting and treating precancerous and pre-invasive cancerous lesions; reducing the risk of myocardial infarction by lowering high blood pressure or controlling diabetes mellitus; reducing the adverse effects of diarrhoea in children by training parents and community health workers to administer oral rehydration solutions.
- Tertiary prevention aims to limit the damage caused by established disease and to optimize the quality of life of those affected. An exercise and training programme to help a stroke victim regain speech, cognitive, or motor functions would be an example of tertiary prevention.

Primary, secondary, and tertiary prevention overlap, and distinctions between levels of prevention are useful but not precise. The term "prevention" is used here in a broad sense, to encompass all three levels, and thus includes curative and rehabilitative as well as primary preventive activities.

Use of screening in preventive health services

In populations known to have a high prevalence of certain infectious diseases, including diseases with asymptomatic phases, early detection and treatment are widely recognized to be a useful adjunct to broader measures aimed at primary prevention. Such broader measures might include improvements in socioeconomic status, education, nutrition, environmental conditions and, in some cases, immunization (McKeown & Lowe, 1974; Terris, 1981; Roemer, 1984).

The screening of all pregnant women to detect and intervene early with risks to their own and their children's health has been shown to be associated with improved health status among high-risk populations, when coupled with the promotion of breast-feeding, birth-spacing, and adequate maternal nutrition (CTF, 1984; Institute of Medicine, 1985, 1988; Royston & Armstrong, 1989). Questions remain about the optimal number and timing of prenatal visits for different risk groups (WHO, 1985a), the optimal content of prenatal care (Institute of Medicine, 1988), and the relative importance of social support as compared with medical care (Phaff, 1986). It is difficult to specify the exact contribution made by prenatal screening itself, because it cannot be separated from the promotional and medical care services into which it is integrated. Isolating the effects of prenatal screening is also rendered difficult by the fact that changes in socioeconomic conditions have tended to accompany the introduction or expansion of prenatal and neonatal care programmes that have included screening (Chamberlain, 1984).

The periodic screening of children's growth and development within programmes providing immunization and other components of well-child care has been an established practice in many developing and industrialized countries for decades. The timing of immunizations has provided a convenient schedule for most activities of health screening in children; in fact, such screening has at times been viewed as a means of ensuring the completion of immunization schedules. However, there has been widespread concern about the general applicability of physical growth standards across diverse populations. Furthermore, questions have been raised about the appropriateness of growth monitoring of children under conditions — e.g., of widespread malnutrition due to community-wide inadequate food supply — where health services have little or nothing to offer families whose children show poor growth, except to stimulate parental guilt and anxiety. The clinical significance of some commonly screened-for conditions has been questioned (USPSTF, 1989). And there are doubts about common screening practices for

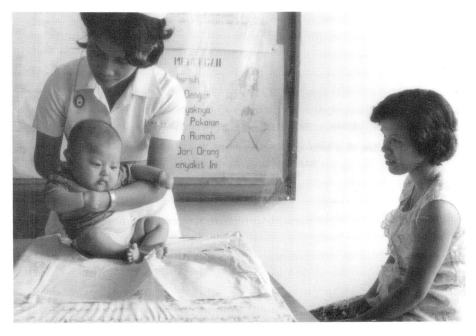

The periodic screening of children's growth and development within programmes providing immunization and other components of well-child care is an established practice in many countries. Examination of an infant in a well-baby programme in Malaysia. (WHO/17411)

conditions of questionable treatability or for which the available test is of doubtful accuracy, for example mild to moderate scoliosis (Chamberlain, 1984; CTF, 1984; Li et al., 1985). Recent publications from the United Kingdom recommend placing greater reliance on explicit enquiry by practitioners regarding any parental concern, rather than subjecting all children to a number of common screening procedures (Hall, 1989; Macfarlane et al., 1989). Such an approach to early detection relies on parents having knowledge of children's normal behaviour and appearance, and on good communication between health care providers, patients, and families.

Routine population-based health screening is best established in maternal and child health programmes, i.e., in prenatal care and well child care (Chamberlain, 1984). In addition, there have been well documented successes, in all age groups, with the early detection and treatment of certain diseases or their precursors that may have prolonged asymptomatic phases. Examples include screening for sexually transmitted diseases, tuberculosis (Mountin, 1950), and certain non-infectious diseases primarily affecting adults; cancer of the uterine cervix in women at high risk (Pinotti et al., 1981; Sampaio Goes, 1981; Tao et al., 1984; Yang et al., 1985; Shrivastav et al., 1986; Stanley et al., 1987); breast cancer in women aged 50 and above (Morrison, 1986); and oral cancer in places where treatment is available locally (Warnakulasuriya et al., 1983, 1984; WHO Meeting, 1984).

In many countries since the 1960s, mass screening for adults has at times been offered as a virtually self-contained service. Automated multiphase testing of adults with batteries of laboratory tests, including chest X-rays, electrocardiograms, and multiple chemical assays of blood and urine, became popular in the USA in the 1960s and 1970s (Chamberlain, 1971; USDHEW, 1971), and is still practised in some places.

However, the effectiveness, in terms of improved health, of multiphase testing in particular and untargeted screening of adults in general has been seriously called into question over the past 25 years in literature from industrialized countries (Nuffield Provincial Hospitals Trust, 1968; Chamberlain, 1971; Frame & Carlson, 1975; CTF, 1979; USPSTF, 1989). Despite this, the general desirability of early detection of occult risk factors, or of presymptomatic or early stages of disease, has gradually come to be widely accepted. The screening of adults for a wide range of risk factors and diseases, especially chronic diseases and cancer, has become standard in many places. It has come to be expected by the educated segments of the population in developing countries as well as in developed countries.

Sophisticated technology for screening has proliferated, and can be a source of substantial earnings for private companies that manufacture, advertise, distribute, maintain, or administer such technology, or that follow-up the results of screening tests. Even without the profit motive, the attraction and power of technology can influence public policy. Decision-makers everywhere are likely to be under strong pressure from a variety of sources to introduce, expand, or maintain screening services. This may be the case even in the absence of adequate scientific evidence or of the health service infrastructure needed to guarantee that screening will result in improved health, especially for those in greatest need.

Unfortunately, low cost per person screened (e.g., in the case of measuring blood pressure) has sometimes been used to justify the use of screening. The cost of definitive diagnosis and the total cost of effective intervention to address the risks identified by screening are often not sufficiently considered; and the total cost is often not weighed against the cost of an alternative approach, not involving screening, that may be more effective. Adverse effects on individuals, such as medical complications arising from screening or diagnostic tests or from the interventions, unnecessary anxiety, loss of privacy, or social stigmatization, are often not taken sufficiently into account. The overall social costs of decisions on the allocation of resources are often especially neglected.

Reassessing the value of the early detection of asymptomatic health conditions

In the light of accumulating evidence, and with increasing attention being paid to considerations of cost-containment, the possibility that untargeted health screening can be wasteful is arousing increasing concern in developed countries (Frame & Carlson, 1975; CTF, 1979, 1984, 1986; USPSTF, 1989). The current reassessment in this area is largely due to the meticulous and exhaustive work of the Canadian Task Force on the Periodic Health Examination, which was first published in 1979 and has been updated several times since. The US Preventive Services Task Force published a report in 1989 reviewing more recent evidence but using criteria similar to those used by the Canadian Task Force for assessing preventive services. Both task forces concluded that many screening practices commonly performed in adults and some commonly performed in children are not justified by the scientific evidence on the efficacy of the tests or the effectiveness of early intervention. Guidelines on screening children published in 1989 in the United Kingdom recommend the discontinuation of many tests that are currently widely performed, primarily because of doubts about their effectiveness (Hall, 1989; Macfarlane et al., 1989).

Concern has been expressed in many studies about the potentially harmful effects of untargeted screening when false positives can generate significant anxiety (Halberstam, 1970; Frank & Mai, 1985) even after confirmatory results are negative (Holtzman, 1991). Positive results — whether true or false — may lead to stigmatization with serious social and economic consequences, at times without commensurate benefit to the individual or society. There is also concern about the ethics of screening for health problems where those found to be at risk can be offered no demonstrable benefit (Wilson & Jungner, 1968).

In 1968 WHO published a Public Health Paper entitled *Principles and practice of screening for disease*, as a point of reference for developing as well as developed countries (Wilson & Jungner, 1968). This was followed by working papers for the technical discussions on mass health examinations, held on the occasion of the Twenty-fourth World Health Assembly in 1971, in which Member States commented on their experiences with routine screening (WHO, 1971; Wilson, 1971). These discussions focused particularly on public health screening efforts covering large population groups. A consensus seemed to emerge from these discussions that great caution should be exercised regarding the adoption of untargeted screening activities for adults, especially in developing countries.

Since then, however, the theoretical and practical issues that arose in the World Health Assembly's discussions on mass health examinations have not been addressed in a systematic fashion at the international level. Moreover, landmark documents on screening in developed countries have been produced in the last 15 years; these documents are known to many policy-makers and have been influential in developing as well as developed countries (CTF, 1979; USPSTF, 1989; Hall, 1989; Holland & Stewart, 1990). The health transition, described earlier, has by now affected most developing countries, which currently have morbidity and mortality profiles showing a large burden of chronic noncommunicable disease and conditions associated with aging; unfortunately these newer problems are widely accompanied by a continuing high incidence of acute infectious diseases of childhood including conditions preventable by immunization, and excessive maternal morbidity and mortality. Experience with early detection in general and screening in particular has now accumulated in developing countries; this can be helpful in selecting options and orienting policies towards the specific needs of these countries.

The primary health care approach

Since the earlier WHO-initiated discussions on screening in developing countries took place, the principles of primary health care have been formulated. Primary health care is an approach formally enunciated at the Thirty-first World Health Assembly in 1978 as a strategy for achieving the goal of "health for all". The phrase "health for all by the year 2000" is a rallying call signifying the attainment by every person in the world of a certain level of health through access to adequate nutrition, safe water and sanitation, literacy, health education, and basic health services (WHO/UNICEF, 1978). The primary health care approach has led to striking gains in health where it has been applied, even under adverse economic or political conditions that have limited its effects.

The primary health care approach:

- equity
- universal coverage with basic services
- a multisectoral approach (e.g., safe water, sanitation, food supply, education, status of women)
- community involvement
- health promotion

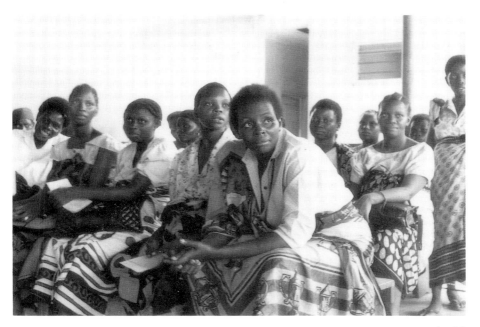

Primary health care uses a multisectoral approach that recognizes the importance to health of education, promoting the status of women and overall socioeconomic development.

The principles of primary health care may be summarized as:

- a commitment to *equity* in the distribution of resources for health and health care;
- *universal coverage* of a population with the basic preventive and curative services most likely to promote health and prevent or control disease; these comprise primary and secondary levels of medical care as well as a wide range of other health-promoting services;
- a *multisectoral approach* that recognizes the importance of education, nutrition, sanitation, and other environmental conditions, as well as the role of the status of women and overall socioeconomic development, in health and illness;
- the promotion of *community involvement* in health activities, not only because of its potential for achieving results at lower cost but because of its relevance for the empowerment of communities and thus for long-term social development;
- an emphasis on the *promotion of health* and not merely the absence of disease.

Primary health care includes, but is more than, primary medical care, a term that has been in use for a longer period of time. Primary medical care (often referred to simply as primary care) denotes only a level of the health care delivery system, i.e., the first-contact level, at which nonspecialized personnel provide basic care for the most common health problems; patients may then be referred to the secondary or tertiary levels (see Glossary) if indicated. By contrast, primary health care is a complex multifaceted approach in which an emphasis on solving problems at the primary medical care level is only one component, along with prevention and alleviation of health problems through nonmedical interventions. While the primary level of medical care is emphasized, both secondary and tertiary care should also be available within a primary health care system on referral from the primary care level, allocated according to need as resources permit. Primary health care should not mean "poor care for poor people"; it is rather a strategy for making the most efficient and most equitable use of limited resources to improve health within a broad sociopolitical strategy for the benefit of the entire society. Primary health care is a health-focused development strategy.

The primary health care approach addresses the health needs of the entire population, and does not just provide care for current users of the available clinical services. Primary health care is, thus, essentially population-based. Moreover, it implies activities far beyond the limited scope of medical services, for example, in such sectors as education, nutrition, sanitation and water supply, and overall community development. At its most developed level,

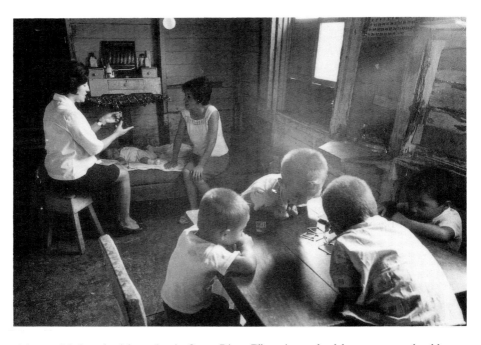

A home visit by a health worker in Costa Rica. The primary health care approach addresses the healh needs of the entire population, and does not just provide care for current users of the available clinical services. (P. Almasy/WHO/15541)

primary health care also implies the active participation of the target population in designing and evaluating their health services.

> Primary health care is intrinsically population-based, i.e., focused on the needs of whole populations, and community-oriented, rather than concerned principally with the current users of clinical services who may not represent the segments of the population in greatest need.

Valuable experience has accrued over the past two decades in the application of the primary health care approach as a means of achieving health for all, despite formidable obstacles. In the light of this experience, and with the principles of primary health care as a point of reference, the appropriate use of health screening now needs to be reassessed.

The role of population-based screening within primary health care

Screening is a potentially useful tool within a primary health care strategy. In line with the primary health care principle of equity, screening can be thought of as a way of identifying those in greatest need of particular interventions to promote health or prevent disease. In this sense, it is a tool for guiding decisions on resource allocation. But this purpose is served only when screening activities are population-based, i.e., focused on populations and subpopulations known from prior studies to be at the greatest risk of having the particular health problems that are being sought and in greatest need of the measures available to address them.

Low socioeconomic status is closely associated with an increased risk of disease and poor health for numerous reasons, including poor nutritional status, exposure to environmental hazards in homes and workplaces, and limited access to health services. Certain population groups may be at particularly high risk, for example, migrant farm labourers, refugees and other immigrants, and urban slum dwellers. Within a given community, particular households or families will be at higher risk and may require screening with greater frequency, or for more conditions, than other households. With a population-based approach, priority would be given to outreach activities directed at high-risk subpopulations. Population-based screening requires at least a basic knowledge of the distribution of levels of general socioeconomic and environmental risk across subpopulations; of basic indicators of health status; and of the accessibility of health services. Such information might be quantitative or qualitative, and ideally would be both.

It would obviously be convenient to offer a screening service first to those segments of the population already using existing services for other purposes; such persons are most likely to understand the value of preventive services for asymptomatic conditions and least likely to require special efforts to reach. Such non-population-based screening activities — i.e., screening activities performed within clinical facilities for current users of those facilities, in the absence of carefully designed outreach efforts to guarantee that those at greatest risk are screened and receive the benefits of appropriate follow-up — are likely to aggravate existing inequities and are not consistent with the primary health care approach. This notion is discussed in more detail later in this chapter. Methods for identifying the subpopulations likely to benefit most from screening-and-timely-intervention activities are discussed in Chapter 3.

Preconditions for successful screening

The primary health care approach prompts the following question: Especially in developing countries, could the resources expended on screening activities be better used for preventive or curative efforts that do not depend on screening? In any country, but perhaps especially in developing countries, health screening activities could tend to divert attention from efforts at primary prevention of the most important causes of poor health, or from universal coverage with basic curative services. This is especially true when primary prevention and universal coverage present significant challenges at the policy level and when the costs of the screening activity appear low because it is mistakenly viewed in isolation from the overall strategy required to make it useful.

Throughout the world, success with screening has depended on the existence of certain prior conditions, primarily information on which segments of the population are at greatest risk, and the will and resources to reach the segments of the population in greatest need. Other preconditions include education of the public and health workers, and an adequate infrastructure for the organization of services, not only for testing, but for the follow-up and treatment of persons with abnormal results. This requires an information and communication system capable of ensuring referrals between different levels of care when necessary in following up abnormal findings. It also requires a sufficient level of technological development to provide effective treatment for those at highest risk. These preconditions are often not met for large segments of the population in developing countries in respect of many conditions for which screening is widely used in more affluent settings. Chapter 2 presents criteria for deciding whether or not to use screening to deal with a given problem.

Commitment to primary health care raises other issues that may not arise within a purely scientific or technical framework or from an ethical perspective centred only on the individual. At times, screening may be aimed at diseases whose control or cure requires a high level of technology currently out of the reach of local resources. This is likely to divert efforts from the resolution of problems at the primary care or community level. An investment at the primary care or primary prevention level might have a far greater chance of successful implementation in the short term and make a much greater contribution to long-term social progress, than would allocation of resources to activities involving screening.

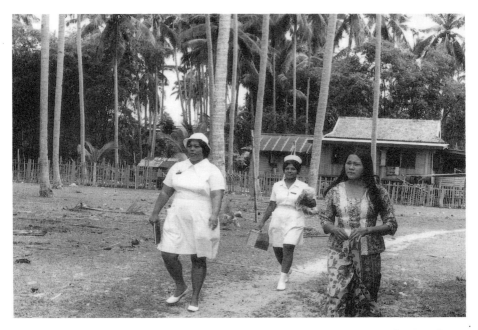

Health workers in Malaysia arriving at a village with no permanently staffed health care facility. Outreach and follow-up on screening results may be especially difficult in some areas, and development of the basic health system infrastructure may be necessary before screening can be used successfully. (WHO/17412)

Furthermore, especially in the developing countries, those in greatest need may not have access to even the most basic curative services; these persons would be unlikely to seek services in the absence of symptoms. Those most likely to seek or be offered screening are generally the more educated segments of society, with the easiest access to health services. Such persons are also most likely to insist on a definitive diagnosis and appropriate treatment for any potential problems detected by screening. Thus, if new technology is introduced for definitive diagnosis or cure, the benefits are likely to be reaped only, or primarily, by a small proportion of the population, not necessarily those in greatest need. Where resources are extremely limited, fewer resources could then be available for reaching the most underserved groups with basic services in their communities. Thus, the premature introduction of screening could unintentionally serve to exacerbate inequities by directing additional resources towards the more privileged segments of the population.

> When the entire population is not yet adequately covered with basic preventive and curative services, screening activities will tend to increase inequities in the distribution of resources for health: the most privileged segments of society — those who already have the best access to health services — are most likely to participate in screening for asymptomatic conditions.

It is important to explore such issues and to share the experience accumulated in various settings. This publication aims to promote the integration of rational population-based preventive practices into long-term comprehensive strategies to strengthen health services and promote health and overall social development. Innovative approaches to the use of screening within community-based programmes have been devised and implemented at the local level in many countries in Africa, Asia, and Latin America. The methods used need to be disseminated and their applicability to other settings considered. Knowledge should be shared about who should be screened for which conditions, how often, by what type of personnel, with what methods, and in what circumstances, with special attention to the needs of developing countries. Developed countries also have much to learn from the creative multisectoral approaches used in developing countries, especially in the light of increasing concern about containing the cost of health care. It is important to note that the availability of a high level of technology does not imply greater equity in the distribution of the resulting benefits; the principles of primary health care thus have much to offer industrialized as well as non-industrialized countries.

When used selectively and with careful planning, health screening can be a powerful tool for the rational targeting of resources for effective and timely intervention. However, extreme caution must be used when considering whether to introduce measures for the early detection of asymptomatic conditions — i.e., screening — into routine health services.

When the preconditions for primary prevention are not shared by the population as a whole and the infrastructure for basic curative services is inadequate to cover the entire population, introduction of screening may exacerbate inequities and retard long-term social development. Alternative approaches that do not involve screening — typically, those directed at primary prevention and at providing universal access to basic services — may be preferable. In general, where primary prevention is possible, it should have priority over approaches involving health screening that seek to minimize health damage but do not eliminate its root causes.

CHAPTER 2

Deciding whether or not to use screening in a primary health care context

Before implementing any services involving screening, careful consideration must be given to the question whether or not it is advisable to use screening at that particular time under the prevailing conditions, or whether other strategies might be preferable. The criteria listed below should be applied systematically in decision-making on whether to use screening. The first four criteria are drawn primarily from the work of Wilson & Jungner (1968); the work of the Canadian Task Force on the Periodic Health Examination (CTF, 1979) and the US Preventive Services Task Force (USPSTF, 1989) was also helpful in formulating the first four criteria. The three final criteria have been added because of their importance from the standpoint of primary health care. The criteria should be considered in the order in which they are presented.

Seven criteria for deciding whether or not to use health screening

1. Is the condition to be detected of public health importance?
2. Are there effective preventive or curative measures to deal with the condition when it is detected at an early stage?
3. Is there a safe, ethical, and efficacious procedure for detecting the condition at a sufficiently early stage to permit effective intervention?
4. Are the screening procedures, definitive diagnosis, and the appropriate interventions acceptable to the population?
5. Is it feasible to carry out the relevant screening, diagnostic, and timely intervention practices in a population-based fashion with existing resources or with resources that could be obtained during the planning period, given sufficient political will?
6. Will the adoption and implementation of the screening, diagnostic, and timely intervention practices strengthen development of the health system and overall societal development, in a manner consistent with primary health care principles?
7. Is the cost of the screening-and-timely-intervention efforts warranted, given all the considerations in items 1–6 above and in comparison with alternative uses of the resources?

---

1. Is the condition to be detected of public health importance?

The burden of suffering that the condition represents for the society should be large enough to warrant special effort. Priority should be given to conditions having a significant impact on the quality of life and survival of a large proportion of the population. Devastating but rare conditions should receive attention only after common causes of significant suffering or disability have been dealt with.

2. *Are there effective preventive or curative measures to deal with the condition when it is detected at an early stage?*

Effective intervention may be carried out wholly or primarily within the health sector, may require intersectoral coordination, or may depend largely on action in other sectors, e.g., agriculture. It may require action at the policy or programme level, involve community mobilization, or consist primarily of clinical treatment of individuals. In some cases, there is no benefit to be derived from intervening before symptoms occur.

3. *Is there a safe, ethical, and efficacious method for detecting the condition at a sufficiently early stage to permit effective intervention?*

Effective screening for some conditions may require invasive tests with risks that outweigh the potential benefits. The early detection of some problems or the appropriate follow-up of screening results may require methods that violate ethical principles, such as a person's right to autonomy, privacy, and confidentiality. If there is no safe and ethical method of screening and timely intervention, the possibility of using screening should be rejected and alternative approaches should be developed to address the problem. Legal and ethical issues are discussed further in Chapter 3.

The screening procedure must be accurate (both sensitive, i.e., with relatively few false negatives, and specific, i.e., with relatively few false positives) and reliable (yielding reproducible results). It should have good positive and negative predictive values in the population to be screened (see Glossary). Certain screening procedures that have high predictive values in particular groups may have poor predictive values in others. For example, mammography is an excellent tool for screening women over 50 years of age for breast cancer, but appears to be a poor screening test in younger women (see page 134).

If criteria 1–3 are met, the following questions should then be asked.

4. *Are the screening and definitive diagnosis procedures and the appropriate interventions acceptable to the population in need of the services?*

Screening or diagnostic procedures or treatments that are inconvenient, uncomfortable, or invasive, violate cultural taboos, or result in social stigmatization or economic hardship are likely to be insufficiently used by the public. The best way to avoid introducing unacceptable services is to involve members

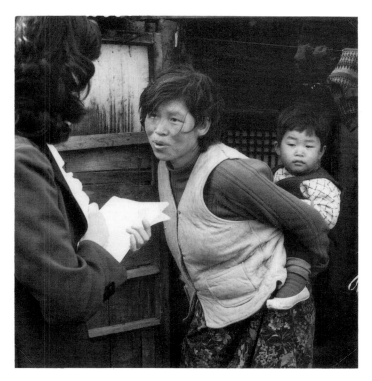

Assessing the acceptability of services: a Korean woman is interviewed about her needs and preferences for family planning services. (P. Almasy/WHO/16398)

of the community in decisions about which services, if any, to introduce, and how. The preferences and convenience of the population to be screened and treated on the basis of screening results are frequently not considered, with predictable consequences. For example, workers need preventive services they can receive without loss of pay. Maternal and child health services, including family planning, need to be organized so as to take account of problems of child care, transport, and the responsibilities of working mothers. The maximum integration of screening activities into established, locally available services used by the population will tend to minimize inconvenience.

Attention to cultural preferences is essential. For example, it may be important for gynaecological and obstetric services to be provided by women only; in some cultures, all services to women need to be provided by women. Blood-testing may not be acceptable in some societies. Health workers involved in early detection activities need to be trained to encourage the use of services by explaining the process to patients, by providing the services in a courteous and considerate manner, and by respecting patients' privacy. Intensive retraining and periodic refresher courses may be necessary to foster the appropriate attitude towards patients. In small communities where workers and patients know each other well, special training and appropriate systems of documentation and handling information should be developed to ensure the confidentiality of potentially sensitive data; periodic retraining is essential.

Even services that are acceptable may not be used if they are not valued by the population. Public education may be necessary, with special outreach to groups at particularly high risk. Community involvement in the design, implementation, and evaluation of services can help ensure that they are acceptable to, valued, and hence used by those in need.

5. Is it feasible to carry out the relevant screening, diagnostic, and timely intervention procedures in a population-based fashion with existing resources or with resources that could be obtained during the planning period, given sufficient political will?

To answer this question, it is necessary to estimate the total resources and costs involved in screening, diagnosis, and effective intervention. The estimate will be based in part on the direct and indirect costs of each screening procedure, multiplied by the estimated number of persons to be screened. This includes the initial investment required to put in place the capacity to perform screening, as well as the recurrent costs of performing each screening procedure. Indirect costs are difficult to calculate, but should include at least the costs of the required planning, public education, and staff training.

Costs also include the costs of definitive diagnosis, based on the estimated number of people who will have abnormal results on screening, and the direct and indirect costs of performing the relevant confirmatory tests, as well as expenses for transport, record-keeping, and communication.

The estimate of the costs of treatment should be based on the number of persons who are expected to need treatment, and should include the costs of long-term follow-up activities; such costs may be considerable, as in the case of the control of high blood pressure. For many health risks, such as asymptomatic high blood pressure, short-term intervention at the individual level is unlikely to be worth while unless it is accompanied by long-term follow-up; it is inappropriate to implement blood pressure screening until such long-term follow-up for those in greatest need can be ensured.

Reaching the population at greatest risk will often depend on involving members of the population as active promoters of the effort. The costs associated with outreach and community involvement are legitimate components of a screening budget and should be taken into account in feasibility studies.

Special costs must be considered in special settings. For example, the costs of screening and ensuring follow-up for nomadic populations may greatly exceed those for sedentary populations (Imperato et al., 1973). In one area of Nepal, local feasibility studies led to the conclusion that the lack of X-ray centres, qualified technicians, and doctors able to interpret radiographs meant that tuberculosis case-finding by sputum microscopy, "implemented by auxiliary

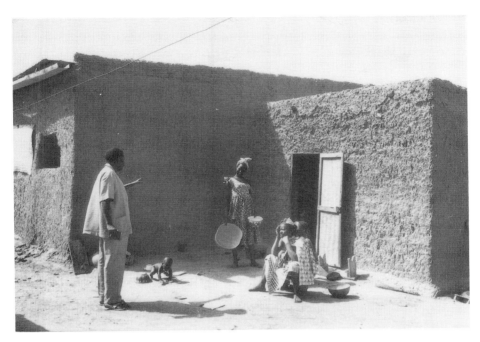

Is it feasible to reach the population at greatest risk? A neighbourhood outreach worker in Mali encourages people to come for early detection of onchocerciasis. (WHO/9952)

health workers ... [with] ... adequate training and long-term support" was the most suitable method for tuberculosis screening (Peresra, 1978).

It must be possible to apply the method in a population-based fashion; it is not sufficient to offer the detection procedure and the relevant follow-up measures only to those already receiving care for other reasons. The service must aim eventually to reach the entire population at substantial risk; initially, services may be targeted to those at the very highest risk and later expanded, as resources permit, to those at lower but still significant levels of risk. It is essential that services should be targeted according to the known distribution of risk in the entire population and not according to the convenience of health care providers or the demands of the more privileged sectors of society. The targeting of screening services is discussed further in Chapter 3.

It may not be feasible to use screening at a particular time because of a lack of resources for the proper implementation of the entire strategy of screening, diagnosis, and timely intervention. However, consideration of all seven criteria may lead to the conclusion that it would be highly desirable to implement a given strategy using screening as soon as possible to address a pressing problem. In this case, measures to achieve the necessary preconditions within a specified time frame could be considered; the essential criteria for implementing screening could then be reviewed at a later date. Other approaches could be used in the meantime or might even be preferable in the future.

6. Will the adoption and implementation of the screening, diagnostic, and timely intervention procedures strengthen the development of the health system and overall social development, in a manner consistent with primary health care principles?

Essential questions to ask in considering this criterion are: Will the screening-and-timely-intervention operation tend to increase equity in the allocation of health resources? Is it likely to result in improved health status for those in greatest need? Which population groups are most likely to benefit from screening activities for asymptomatic individuals?

Especially where large population groups, e.g., rural populations, or poor populations on the urban periphery, do not have access to basic health and education services, a decision to conduct screening for an asymptomatic condition is likely to increase disparities between the covered and uncovered populations in terms of the utilization of health services. Screening for asymptomatic conditions is likely to attract the more highly educated, who are also those with greater access to places where screening is performed. Furthermore, screening will result in abnormal findings for some individuals; this will entail additional resources for definitive diagnosis and ultimately for treatment. The screening operation will thus have created a demand among those screened for the provision of additional services. This demand may result in the further allocation of resources that will benefit only a limited number of people who already enjoy better health status and health services than the large underserved groups. Thus, unless services are consciously targeted at those at highest risk, the benefits will generally be enjoyed by those segments of the population that already make most use of health care services. The targeting of screening efforts is discussed further in Chapter 3.

Will the local health system infrastructure tend to be strengthened by the introduction of the activities under consideration? Will there be side benefits such as better coordination between different units or levels within the health system, or between health services and services in other sectors? Will the measures contemplated help to improve the status of women, or will they promote community involvement or contribute in some other way to overall social development? Will they strengthen public awareness of health promotion and prevention?

7. Is the cost of the screening-and-timely-intervention operation warranted, given all the considerations covered in items 1–6 above, in comparison with alternative uses of the resources?

Will the operation divert resources from other measures that are likely to be more effective? What other ways are there of addressing the problem that do not involve screening? Are these better? Will the screening operation divert health workers' attention from more crucial efforts addressing the principal

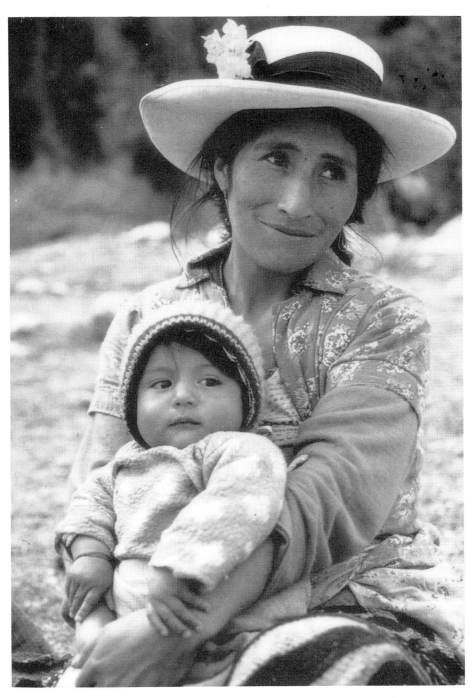

Will the use of screening be consistent with primary health care principles?

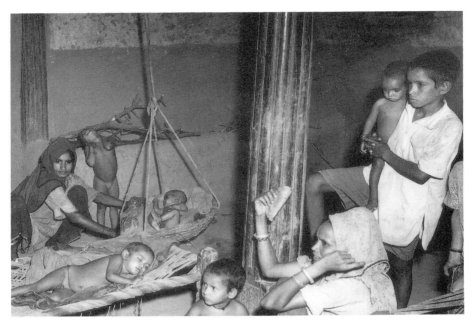

Which population groups are likely to benefit from screening activities for asymptomatic conditions? Will the use of screening tend to increase or decrease equity? (WHO/1579)

health problems of the population? Will it accomplish little but create the impression among the public that their problems are being dealt with and divert their attention from issues of higher priority?

In order to answer these questions, the costs and benefits of the proposed screening and intervention activities must be weighed against those of alternative strategies, taking into account both direct and indirect, as well as immediate and future, benefits (Creese & Parker, 1994).

The best preventive strategy does not always include screening.

When planned thoughtfully and implemented in a population-based fashion, screening can provide a rational basis for resource allocation. It can be used to ensure that preventive measures are applied where they will have the most effect. However, the costs of screening and subsequent follow-up need to be weighed against the savings to be derived from other potentially more effective and efficient uses of resources.

In general, primary prevention is better than a strategy that depends on screening. Especially where an important risk factor can be significantly reduced without medical intervention — as, for example, in the case of smoking — it might be desirable to concentrate the available resources on mass

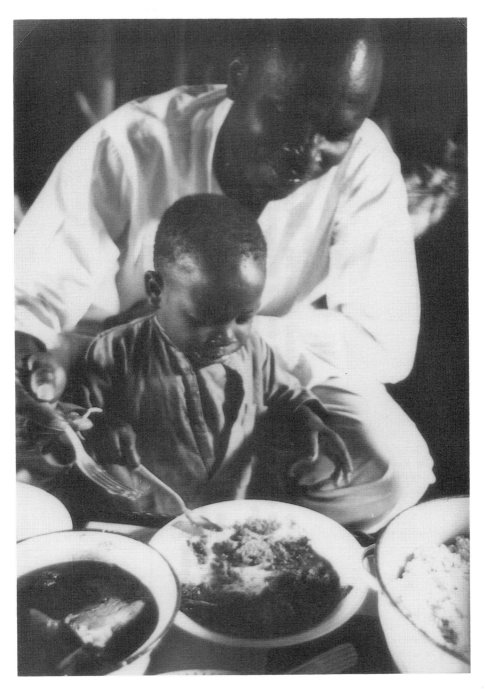

Resources spent on growth monitoring of children may be better spent on health promotion and other action in the community. (WHO/UN/18432)

public education and policy initiatives such as legislation to ban advertising of tobacco products. Even resources spent on growth monitoring of children may, under certain conditions, be better spent on ensuring an adequate food supply at the community level, on community-wide promotional efforts to encourage families to give priority to the nutritional needs of pregnant and lactating women, and children, or on promotion of family planning. In such cases, there might be little to be gained by diverting resources towards a screening operation to identify and treat individuals with the risk factor.

In some situations it may be preferable to mount a mass public education campaign to encourage those with a given risk factor, symptom, or sign to consult the health services, rather than having health workers go out to find them. The self-referral of symptomatic persons would be followed by appropriate diagnostic tests and accompanied by case-finding activities covering persons consulting the health services for other reasons. This approach depends on the health services being readily accessible to those at risk, and on a successful mass education effort.

CHAPTER 3

Planning and implementing services using screening in a primary health care context

Planning for services using screening

Once a decision to use screening has been made, on the basis of criteria 1–7 (see Chapter 2), careful planning is required to ensure success. Attention must be paid to certain important issues that frequently arise at the local level in the implementation of services involving screening.[1]

Screening cannot be viewed as a self-contained service. It is a subunit of a process with a multiplicity of components, including the different phases of detection (screening and diagnosis) and of preventive action to respond to the particular problems detected. The planning process needs to cover the selection of locally appropriate methods and criteria and the targeting of services to those in greatest need, as well as education, documentation, preventive intervention, and evaluation. In assessing the costs of a preventive approach

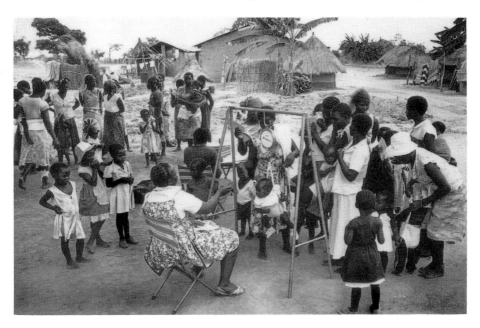

Screening in a well-baby programme in Zimbabwe.   (L. Taylor/WHO/20159)

---

[1] Two helpful general references are: Tarimo & Fowkes, 1989; WHO, 1988.

employing screening, the costs of all these components must be included. The total cost of the entire effort required to achieve improvements in health status needs to be calculated; the cost of the screening component itself may be small compared with the cost of the appropriate follow-up of those screened (see criterion 6, page 26).

Planning needs to encompass administrative as well as financial planning for all activities involved. An adequate administrative infrastructure should be planned for overseeing and coordinating all aspects of the process.

Planning at the local level

There can be large differences between countries, and between provinces, departments, or districts in the same country, in the health problems that are most important. There can also be significant differences in the resources available for priority health problems and sometimes in the most appropriate ways of dealing with them.

Initial planning will be carried out at the national and provincial levels. However, most health activities relevant to primary health care are carried out at the district level and it is at this level that high-priority problems and strategies to address them need to be reassessed and activities planned in detail. Planning at the district level should be based on a review of the high-priority health problems within the district and the resources available to address them in a manner consistent with the values of the population. Representatives of health personnel, of the populations to be screened, and of other sectors whose collaboration will be needed should be actively involved in the planning.

Planning is needed to ensure coordination between the different levels within the local health care system and between the different sectors that will be involved in the screening-diagnosis-and-timely-intervention process. The levels within the district health system that will be involved (community, health post, health centre, district hospital) also need to be considered.

Levels of the district health system to be involved in a screening-diagnosis-and-timely-intervention operation

- The community level (the population itself, volunteers, and traditional healers).
- The peripheral or neighbourhood health post level (sites in rural or peripheral urban areas where basic care is delivered and with no, or only extremely simple, laboratory facilities).
- The health centre level (staffed by salaried health workers, generally including some professionals, usually providing a range of ambulatory services, and capable of performing simple laboratory tests).
- The district hospital level (the central facilities of the district health system, serving as the focus for referrals from the three lower levels, and including inpatient and outpatient services, laboratory and pharmacy facilities, and other district-level referral centres).

Activities should be carried out at the lowest level possible. In general, screening activities should be conducted at the primary care level (i.e., the first-contact level) on an outpatient basis, using nonspecialized personnel. If it is not possible to conduct screening in a primary care facility (community centre, health post, or health centre), primary care personnel should be involved as much as possible, partly to ensure continuity of care and partly to strengthen primary care services.

Selection of locally appropriate methods and criteria

The methods used to screen for a specified problem or risk factor should reach the entire population at risk, be sufficiently accurate and reliable, have good predictive value, and be safe and acceptable to the population and the personnel. They should be consistent with long-term strategies for strengthening health services and promoting overall social development. Here, decisions have to be made about the type of personnel to be involved, whether volunteers, traditional birth attendants, other traditional community healers, salaried health workers, or personnel from other sectors such as teachers. Any early detection method needs to be appropriate to local conditions. A study in an urban area of India concluded that the established method for detecting active leprosy among school-age children — a school survey — was less effective than a neighbourhood-based survey for children living in an urban slum (Soni & Ingle, 1982).

Screening criteria will vary according to local circumstances. For example, a study of screening for fetopelvic dystocia in Zaire concluded that far broader criteria needed to be applied when screening rural women than when screening those living in town, since town-dwellers could be rapidly brought to the referral centre for operative delivery, if necessary (Kasongo Project Team, 1984).

"Method", as used here, also refers to the technique employed for the measurement itself, e.g., verbal enquiry, examination by a trained person without any instruments, the use of simple instruments such as tape measures or scales, or a technique requiring laboratory materials and equipment. Does the method depend on the regular maintenance and restocking of disposable supplies, using resources from outside the district, or will materials always be available within the district? Can the screening be carried out in the community or at the primary care level or does it require the facilities or personnel of a hospital?

Targeting activities for maximum effectiveness

Who should be screened?

Many screening procedures should be carried out for an entire broad population group, e.g., all pregnant women, all infants, all young children, or all women of reproductive age. However, some procedures are appropriate only for specific subpopulations, as defined, for example, by age or special risk factors. Screening, and the associated promotional and preventive efforts, need to be targeted to well defined groups known from prior research to be at elevated risk for the conditions being sought, and likely to be helped by available interventions.

For example, policy concerning the Papanicolaou (Pap) test to detect cancer of the cervix needs to take into account the fact that cervical cancer and precancerous lesions are most prevalent in women over 35 years of age. Efforts at detection should therefore be targeted at that group. Reaching women over 35 presents problems, however, and currently, in most countries, those most likely to receive screening are young women attending family planning clinics, in whom cervical cancer is relatively rare. These younger women have come to expect frequent Pap screening, and if the policy is changed, may feel deprived of what they have come to consider standard care, and anxious about the consequences (see page 131). Another example is the widely applied practice of radiographic screening of whole populations for tuberculosis, which is expensive and often unproductive, even in areas of high prevalence. Case-finding and the promotion of early self-referral can be used to target diagnostic procedures to those with characteristic symptoms, e.g., persistent or productive cough, especially with fever, night sweats, or weight loss. Targeting of re-sources in this way can reduce expense considerably, increase accuracy, and greatly help to reduce the burden of the disease (see page 114).

Multistage screening: disease-specific rapid assessment methods

Multistage screening is a promising approach to the targeting of screening operations. High-risk groups are identified in a first stage, using extremely low-cost methods (e.g., enquiry, questionnaires) that have good sensitivity but may have limited specificity. Persons who test positive are then re-screened using a more specific method and, finally, given a definitive diagnosis. Clearly, the value of such an approach depends on the sensitivity of the methods used in the first stage, and the overall positive and negative predictive values and costs of each screening stage.

An example of a multistage approach is the use of "clinical downstaging" to screen for cervical cancer. Visual examination of the cervix, supplemented by case history, is used to identify the women most in need of cytological testing, in places where an extreme scarcity of resources makes it impossible to screen all women cytologically (see page 131). Another example is the use of a simple questionnaire on gross haematuria to identify groups of schoolchildren at high risk for urinary schistosomiasis; teachers can then use reagent strips to test the children's urine (see page 107).

These and other multistage techniques can also be considered for the preliminary rapid assessment of risk at the community level. Such rapid assessment is usually linked to detection of general socioeconomic and environmental risk. The validation of efficient methods for assessing both disease-specific and general socioeconomic risks should have high priority on a research agenda. A number of recent publications contain valuable information on rapid assessment techniques that could be used for particular disease conditions (Smith, 1989; Vlassof & Tanner, 1992; Lengeler et al., 1991a, b; Manderson & Aaby, 1992).

Preliminary risk assessment at the community level

Screening should be thought of as a tool for directing resources for intervention where they will have the greatest impact. To do this, screening itself must be carefully targeted and based on adequate prior knowledge of the general social, economic, and environmental conditions in a community. Such knowledge will often determine the frequency of screening or early detection and the techniques to be used. For example, door-to-door surveys of the immunization status of preschool-age children may be unnecessary in relatively affluent neighbourhoods, but helpful when performed periodically in poor urban and rural neighbourhoods, especially if immunizations are readily available at the time of the survey.

A system for classifying the overall socioeconomic and environmental risks to communities and households has been used by the public health ministries in Costa Rica and Cuba. Different schedules are used for the routine surveillance of environmental conditions, the immunization status of preschool-age children, and the number of pregnant women receiving prenatal care. Neighbourhood and household visits are made by primary health care workers. Those at highest risk receive more frequent and intensive surveillance and support, including household visits where appropriate. In Costa Rica, the communities at lowest risk on the initial screening may be deemed not to need assessment at the household level, or it may be decided to assess them less frequently or less intensively. In Cuba, the "family doctor" approach means that a physician is responsible for the health care of all families living within a defined geographical area and is expected to visit homes regularly. This makes it possible for the individual physician to know the general risk level in a community, in subgroups within that community, and in individual families.

Locally appropriate schemes may be developed to classify general risk levels for communities and families. Appropriate indicators of risk may be quite simple: for example, health programme managers in an area of Sri Lanka found that communities that had fewer than a certain number of coconut trees per population were at significantly higher risk of a number of health problems, and that this criterion (which correlated well with socioeconomic level in the area) could be used to direct resources. Rapid assessment methods, as well as all screening procedures, need to be validated and their sensitivity, specificity, and predictive values determined.

Frequency of screening

Determining the frequency of screening requires a knowledge of the natural history, including the duration of latency, of the conditions to be detected. For example, in most countries, cervical cancer screening with Pap smears is carried out more frequently than is rational (typically, annually) for low-risk women using family planning programmes, who are generally quite young, while the women at highest risk (those over 35 years of age, who are less likely to be using family planning services) often go entirely unscreened. Women who have had one normal Pap test and who are not at special risk can be screened far less frequently; the resources thus saved can be used for special outreach activities targeting high-risk women. Higher-risk populations may need to be screened more frequently (see page 131).

To consider another example: in low-risk populations it may be sufficient to screen all children for immunization status on starting school and at scheduled well-baby or well-child visits. But, among socioeconomically vulnerable groups or in areas with poor access to health services, there may be a need for periodic neighbourhood-based screening of infants, preschool-age children, and children of school age who do not attend school, to check immunization status and look for other conditions reviewed in Chapters 6 and 7.

Integration of screening into existing services

It is preferable to integrate screening activities and the necessary follow-up into existing health and social service programmes, rather than have separate

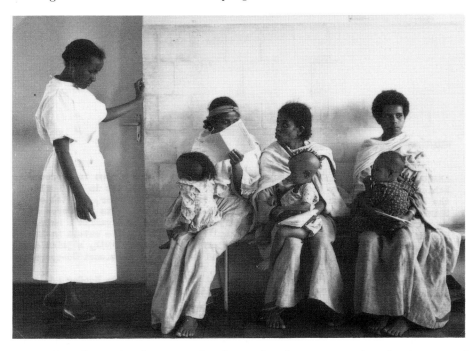

Integration of screening into comprehensive services is more convenient for the users of services and permits health workers to get to know people in a broader, family-oriented context. (WHO/8929)

services for screening or disease-specific programmes. In some cases, a separate, one-off early detection and follow-up campaign may be appropriate, e.g., as a pilot effort, but ideally early detection including screening should be part of continuous, coordinated, and integrated programme activities. The sustainability of a screening-and-timely-intervention operation needs to be considered. As much as possible, high-risk groups should be reached through existing programme structures rather than through the creation of new and separate programmes. Where possible, screening for a variety of conditions affecting a given population group should be carried out at the same time and along with appropriate health promotional activities by primary care personnel, as is standard practice in prenatal care and well-child care programmes.

Integration of screening into ongoing primary care services will greatly facilitate effective follow-up. Primary care personnel are likely to know the people in their community and should thus be able to locate an individual with positive screening results. Experienced primary care personnel should also be able to help formulate a realistic plan for preventive intervention based on the risks detected and to encourage individuals, families, and the community to take appropriate action. A population-based programme that is well integrated into primary care can be used to identify other people who need special attention. For example, a well-child programme caring for one child in a particular family can identify other children, pregnant women, or women of reproductive age in that family who are likely to be inadequately immunized, or identify a family at generally increased risk for social or economic reasons.

Intersectoral coordination

During the planning phase, the following questions need to be considered: Which institutions outside the health sector should be involved — schools, agricultural associations, trade unions, employers, community organizations, transport, communication, or other governmental or nongovernmental services? How and where will the appropriate preventive measures be carried out?

Education

The planning and implementation of any system of screening, diagnosis, and timely intervention involves two educational components: (1) initial training and continuing education of health workers at all levels (including those involved in record-keeping); and (2) education of the public through the media and community organizations. Public education can also be carried out by providers of health or social services or through providing promotional material at the institutions offering such services. However, this will only reach those already using the services, who may not be the target population that should be given priority. Public education is necessary so that those at risk will not only tolerate but will actively seek the appropriate preventive services. A study in India demonstrated that, in areas with a high prevalence of leprosy,

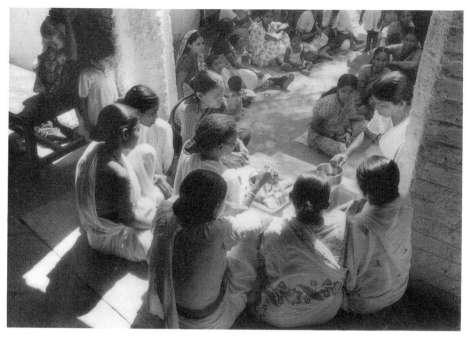

Costs of training need to be considered in planning screening activities: training traditional birth attendants in south India. (WHO/6248)

mass public education, combined with training of health workers, is accompanied by marked increases in the number of cases detected, which may make mass screening of asymptomatic persons unnecessary (Ganapati et al., 1984).

Intensive public education is especially important when new practices are being introduced, and among segments of the population with less access to services than others. It should cover: the value of screening or other forms of early detection; indications for screening (e.g., for pregnant women, for infants and preschool children, and for persons presenting certain risk factors); conditions screened for (e.g., sexually transmitted diseases, cancer, or chronic diseases); and the places where appropriate services are available. The need to teach health workers the importance of courtesy and confidentiality in order to increase the acceptability of preventive services was discussed briefly in Chapter 2. Health workers also need to be trained in how to tell people that they have a positive test result; if adequate counselling cannot be provided to persons testing positive, then the health care system is not ready to introduce screening. Screening for HIV infection, in particular, requires skilled counselling. The counselling required to accompany genetic screening is extremely sophisticated and needs more advanced training than is generally available at the primary care level.

If people are to make appropriate use of screening services and comply with follow-up recommendations, they need to understand why the screening is being performed. Because social support may be crucial in ensuring screening and follow-up for those who need it, it is not enough simply for patients to receive instructions from health care providers. For example, a pregnant woman whose work in the fields is economically important for her family may not be able to attend a prenatal clinic if her family does not accept the importance of such care. Families and communities need to be educated so that they will accept and encourage the allocation of time and resources to the screening and appropriate follow-up of vulnerable persons, e.g., pregnant women, children, and the elderly.

Documentation for following up individuals, families, and communities

---

Information infrastructure needed for any screening operation

In any screening operation, an adequate information infrastructure is needed:

1. for patient tracking, i.e., to provide appropriate follow-up for conditions detected in individuals;
2. for quality assurance;
3. to protect confidentiality;
4. to evaluate the process and results of screening and timely intervention efforts in order to determine whether these efforts should be continued and for which population groups;
5. if possible, to ensure that the information gained from screening makes the greatest possible contribution to information for programme planning and population monitoring.

The documentation needed for patient tracking consists of the minimum information required to follow up on abnormal results. One of the most frequent errors that occurs when resources are very limited is to provide the resources needed to conduct the actual screening but to allocate insufficient resources to collect the information needed for effective follow-up. If documentation and, consequently, the follow-up are inadequate, screening will be of no benefit.

The identification of patients with abnormal results in screening tests is often incomplete or incorrect. People may use different names, may move frequently, or may give incorrect or incomplete addresses. Mistakes may be made in recording names or addresses, rendering follow-up impossible. If the persons screened are not known personally to the health workers responsible for follow-up, it can be useful to ask for an alternative address (e.g., of the place of work or of family or friends residing elsewhere) at the time a test is performed. Careful attention must be given to protecting the confidentiality of the results of screening or diagnostic tests (see page 40).

Sometimes the documentation needed for screening-and-timely-intervention activities may contain information useful for monitoring health needs at the community level. Examples include the proportion of two-year-olds adequately immunized and the proportion of pregnant women testing positive for sexually transmitted diseases. For the purpose of population monitoring, information should be reported as an aggregate, with all personal identifiers removed.

Evaluation

Systematic evaluation is needed of screening-and-timely-intervention operations and their end results, for the following purposes: (1) as a basis for decisions on future resource allocation; (2) as a means of quality assurance, e.g., to find out whether screening results were followed up, definitive diagnostic tests performed, and appropriate treatments given; and (3) as a source of information for feedback to health workers and to the population. The involvement of both the community and health workers at different levels should be sought in evaluating the implementation of services. Feedback is needed on both the process and the end results to motivate health workers to promote quality. Information on results can also help motivate the public, and promote improved or continuing use of services and preventive practices on a community and individual level.

The evaluation of end results may include an assessment of side benefits; this should not, however, be a substitute for the assessment of results against the central goals of screening-and-intervention operations. For example, a side benefit of screening may be that health workers become more alert to opportunities for timely intervention in general, and thus provide better care. However, such side benefits do not justify a strategy involving screening if there is no demonstrable direct effect or if the total benefits are not commensurate with the resources required, in comparison with alternative options.

Legal and ethical issues

Difficult legal and ethical issues can arise in carrying out screening and follow-up activities; these important issues are only briefly summarized here. The most obvious potential ethical dilemmas are those arising when conditions being screened for are likely to cause people testing positive to suffer social stigmatization, loss of income or employment, or legal consequences (Wilson & Jungner, 1968; USPSTF, 1989). Screening for HIV infection is a particularly dramatic case in point, in view of the current worldwide epidemic. Because screening for HIV illustrates many important legal and ethical issues with wide applicability, many examples are drawn from that area. Similar issues arose earlier in this century in connection with tuberculosis and other infectious diseases and are relevant when considering screening for any condition. Many important legal and ethical issues applicable to screening in general are discussed by Gunderson et al. (1989) and in a WHO publication on genetic screening (Modell et al., 1991). A WHO document on HIV testing is reproduced in Annex 1; most of the issues it addresses have wide applicability to screening for other conditions.

Notions of privacy and related ethical obligations and legal requirements may vary from society to society. However, the right to privacy (Gunderson et al., 1989), as defined by the culture of the population to be screened, must be respected and taken into account as a fundamental human right when any

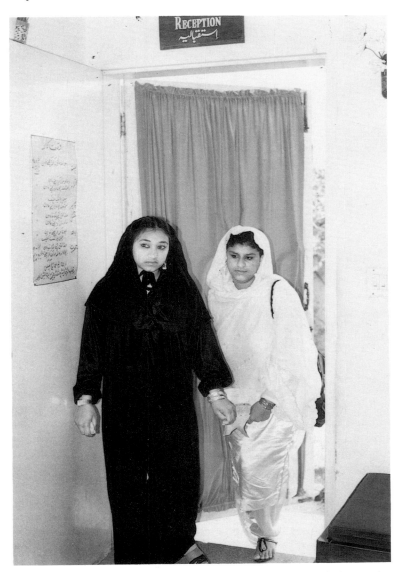

The right to privacy, as defined by the culture of the population to be screened, must be respected when planning and implementing screening activities.

health services, including those involving screening, are being designed. Mechanisms are needed to ensure confidentiality at all stages of a screening-and-timely-intervention operation, while providing adequate information for following up individuals found positive and their contacts. Before any screening is instituted, it should be ascertained to what extent the confidentiality of the records can be ensured. In the context of screening, respecting the right to informed consent means that individuals are adequately informed prior to testing regarding the possible consequences of positive or negative results. In addition to being irrational, involuntary screening is generally unethical and, in many societies, illegal. Perplexing special issues may arise in forensic situations, e.g., screening of a suspected rapist for HIV infection or other sexually transmitted disease in order to provide the information to the victim. Such information will have limited value, however, for example, because of the delay between infection and seroconversion.

Proposals have emerged, and legislation has been considered in certain countries, calling for mandatory HIV testing of health personnel performing procedures involving some possibility of accidental HIV transmission. The argument is that this is necessary in order to protect patients from being infected by health care providers who may not be aware of their condition. Similarly, mandatory HIV testing has been suggested for patients admitted to hospital. However, a reasoned consideration of the practical issues involved shows that such proposals should be rejected. Since some persons with recent infection will not have produced antibodies at the time of testing, it is highly unlikely that mandatory screening of either patients or health workers would be helpful. It would not be possible to determine reliably how frequently to repeat screening, and the costs of repeated screening would be prohibitive.

Furthermore, mandatory testing would result in many people at risk avoiding contact with health services without necessarily changing their high-risk behaviour. Mandatory testing would also consume tremendous resources, and negative results could promote a false sense of security. The available screening tests for HIV infection have a significant false-positive rate and a low positive predictive value in low-risk groups. The risk of the stigmatization of persons detected as positive on screening are so great and the individual and social benefits of mandatory screening so doubtful, that alternative approaches must be considered. A rational alternative is to maintain a voluntary testing policy, while emphasizing education of the public about risk factors and prevention of infection; appropriate precautions should be taken during all procedures involving risk. Intensive public education with community involvement has proved highly effective in preventing HIV transmission. Universal precautions should be taken by health care providers in all areas where HIV is a potential problem — which now means most of the world.

Proposals for the mandatory HIV screening of tourists and immigrants on their entry to a country have been another response motivated by fear rather than by information and reason. These proposals are flawed on practical grounds because of the long period between infection and seroconversion and the low specificity of screening tests, and on ethical grounds because of the harm caused to individuals without benefit to those screened or a clear overriding social benefit. The ethical principle in such situations is that of avoiding doing harm to persons (by labelling them as afflicted with disease), without an overriding social good to be gained from it. The social, economic, and psychological consequences of being labelled HIV-positive are often devastating. The anxiety caused by being labelled as suffering from disease must also be taken into account, especially where a significant proportion of positive screening results are likely to be false positives. The US Preventive Services Task Force was particularly concerned about the harm that screening could cause by erroneous labelling, with consequent anxiety, substantial expenses for definitive diagnosis, and potential social and economic consequences for those labelled (USPSTF, 1989).

Unless a clear and overriding benefit for society at large can be demonstrated, it is also unethical to screen for conditions without ensuring adequate resources for providing effective care for the individuals and communities found to have those conditions. This assumes that the planned and stated purpose of testing is prescriptive screening, rather than epidemiological investigation without identification of individuals. It would thus be unethical to conduct blood-pressure screening in market-places without ensuring that sufficient resources are available for definitive diagnosis and effective long-term treatment of those found to have high blood pressure. Conducting HIV screening without providing effective counselling and support for those with positive test results would also be unethical.

Furthermore, from the primary health care perspective, other important ethical concerns arise with regard to the question of mandatory screening for HIV infection and other conditions. Spending scarce resources on an ineffective approach based on mandatory testing, while neglecting an approach far more likely to be effective, i.e., public education about primary prevention, may violate the ethical principle of doing what is most beneficial for those being cared for. Since the most vulnerable segments of society are those likely to suffer most from lack of information that would help reduce the risk they face, a course of action diverting resources from education to mandatory testing could also potentially violate the ethical principle of distributive justice. This principle is violated by the use of screening when primary prevention, or another approach not depending on screening, would be more beneficial for those sectors of the population in greatest need, and when the use of screening is likely to aggravate existing inequities in the distribution of health services (see Chapter 2).

CHAPTER 4

Development of recommendations on uses of screening in primary health care

The following chapters review options for the use of screening as a primary health care tool to address a number of health problems. The possible use of screening for each of the selected problems is discussed in the light of the criteria and principles presented in Chapters 1–3, with observations on the desirability of screening as compared with other approaches to prevention. We have not attempted to provide technical details on the screening methods, but rather have sought, for each problem, to review the relevance of screening and suggest important general features that would characterize the use of screening within a primary health care strategy. We have also indicated relevant references. It is hoped that the illustrative examples given here will suggest locally appropriate approaches to problems and make the literature more accessible.

In reviewing the literature, we gave priority to reports of experience with screening in developing countries, but references are also included on experience in developed countries that could be of interest elsewhere. Few of the options for using screening that are reviewed have been formally and rigorously validated. It was not within the scope of this publication to evaluate formally the quality of the evidence available on the results of using particular screening methods.

For each health problem or risk factor selected, we generally ask the questions: *Why?* (the rationale for using screening); *Who?* (the groups that should be targeted); *How?* and *When?* These aspects are discussed with reference to experiences recorded in the literature and in the light of the key principles discussed earlier. We then make comments on the level of resources likely to be required for screening, diagnosis, and timely intervention. Finally, a recommendation is made regarding the priority that should be given to the use of screening for the particular problem within a primary health care system, in the light of possible alternative approaches.

One of the key factors in making the recommendations was a consideration of the level of resources required for the screening, diagnosis, and intervention in individuals found to be at elevated risk. Four general levels of resources were distinguished: low, medium, high, and very high.

● **Low.** Procedures requiring a low level of resources can be carried out by enquiry (verbal or questionnaire) or inspection without instruments or laboratory facilities, or with very simple instruments and materials. They do not require professional highly trained staff, and may be performed by a primary health care worker or possibly by a parent or teacher.

● **Medium.** Procedures requiring a medium level of resources involve the basic instruments or laboratory facilities usually found at a health centre, and staff with technical or professional training that is not specialized. Low and medium levels of resources are those used at the primary care level.

● **High.** Procedures requiring a high level of resources use technology that is generally available only at the district or hospital level, or are performed by staff with specialized technical or professional training. This level roughly corresponds to that of secondary care.

● **Very high.** Procedures requiring a very high level of resources involve technology or training that is generally not available at the district or general hospital level, but found only at a national or regional referral centre (tertiary care).

The distinctions between these levels of resources are relative rather than absolute; the more limited the overall resources, the less likely it is that a given level of technology or training will be found at the district or health centre level. Conversely, in a setting where a health system is well developed, relatively sophisticated technology or training may be available at the health centre or even peripheral health post level.

Another key consideration in arriving at the recommendations, in line with the criteria in Chapter 2, was the question whether a more effective means of addressing a given problem without using screening might be preferable. Thus, even if the resources needed for detection and intervention appeared relatively modest, the use of screening was not recommended if an approach not using screening — typically, one emphasizing community-wide primary prevention — appeared more effective and efficient.

For each screening practice reviewed, a recommendation is made on the priority that should be given to its use in a system based on primary health care.

● **"Recommended"** indicates that high priority should be given to considering the screening of asymptomatic persons as part of preventive action aimed at the particular problem or risk factor. In some cases, screening as strictly defined (see Chapter 1 and Glossary) was not deemed appropriate, but early detection of symptoms among persons with unrecognized health problems was recommended. Many important conditions produce characteristic symptoms at a very early stage; these manifestations would be identified as symptoms by persons with a good knowledge of health matters and good access to care, but are likely to go unrecognized by persons with inadequate health knowledge and limited access to care. In such cases, emphasis should be given to large-scale public education and the provision of accessible medical care services so as to promote self-referral for early detection of easily recognizable symptoms.

● **"Not recommended as a priority"** indicates that it is not thought advisable, in a primary health care context, to give priority to an approach using the screening of asymptomatic persons for the particular problem.

● **"Uncertain recommendation"** indicates that existing knowledge is insufficient to justify recommending for or against using the screening of asymptomatic persons as a preventive measure for the particular problem, in a primary health care system. This implies a very strong recommendation to consider a wide range of other alternatives before investing in resources to conduct screening for the problem being considered.

In addition to a recommendation on the appropriateness of screening, attention is called to some priorities for research of relevance to conditions in developing countries. Research priorities may include studies to develop and evaluate cost-effective methods for screening, diagnosis, or timely intervention. The recommendations are listed in the summary tables (pages 139–164) and discussed in Chapters 5–8.

The recommendations are based on the criteria set out in Chapter 2 and on consideration of the reference material accessible for this project. They should not be seen as comparable to the conclusions emerging from the work of the large consensus panels that have undertaken comprehensive and intensive reviews of the subject (see "Introduction"). The recommendations are presented with the hope that they will stimulate discussion, further study, and a consideration of important issues within countries, regions, and districts. They are not meant to argue for or against the use of any particular practice in any particular country; such decisions can only be made after consideration of local conditions.

The list of conditions and practices considered in the following chapters is not exhaustive; it represents an attempt to cover many but certainly not all of the health problems that are important in the developing world and for which screening has been used or should be considered as part of a preventive strategy. It was considered especially important to cover conditions accompanying the health transition. Many important conditions have not been covered or are referred to only briefly. Considerations of space have limited observations, even on those conditions for which there is a rich literature describing and evaluating experience of screening in particular settings. For example, because literature on the detection of tropical diseases is likely to be relatively easily obtainable through other sources, screening for parasitic diseases in developing countries is given very limited treatment in this publication except in a general way, and more emphasis is given to noninfectious diseases. We have also sought to avoid duplicating other up-to-date references, notably those concerning the rapidly evolving field of detection and prevention of HIV infection. Although the criteria and principles put forth in this publication apply to screening in workplaces as well as other settings, it was beyond the scope of this project to deal in detail with special issues that arise with regard to occupational health screening. We have commented on general issues arising in connection with screening for occupational health hazards, but we have not reviewed specific examples. The reader is referred to another WHO publication on this topic (WHO, 1986a).

As the emphasis in this publication is on primary health care, there is little coverage of screening procedures requiring highly specialized tertiary-care resources, since, in many developing countries, it would be beyond the means of the health services to make them available on a population-wide basis. These issues are discussed in the frequently cited review documents on experience in industrialized countries. Low-cost, low-technology options have been emphasized. We have consciously chosen primarily to address the needs and conditions of countries with markedly limited resources that are at present giving priority to achieving universal coverage with basic services for all, rather than providing more expensive services for a few persons unlikely to be at greatest risk.

In the following chapters, screening is discussed in relation to the care of the general population groups targeted by primary health care programmes:

● **Maternal, reproductive/family, and newborn health care (Chapter 5).** This covers programmes for prenatal care, reproductive health care (often called family health care) including family planning, and care of the newborn.

● **Child health care (Chapter 6).** This chapter discusses screening for important problems of infants and children under 6 years of age and screening for problems specific to school-age children, including growth and development, hearing, and vision, and the problems of adolescents, including the risk of teenage pregnancy, sexually transmitted diseases, the use of harmful substances, and violence. While a few infectious diseases of special relevance to children are discussed, infectious diseases that occur in both children and adults are primarily covered in Chapter 7.

● **Care of children and adults to prevent and control communicable diseases (Chapter 7).** Screening in the prevention and control of communicable diseases affecting both children and adults is discussed in this chapter. However, care for children and adults to prevent and control communicable diseases should be integrated into comprehensive primary health care programmes, rather than organized into disease-specific programmes. Special issues regarding infectious diseases among children are covered in Chapter 6 and special issues for adults are addressed in Chapter 8; some communicable diseases are also covered in Chapter 5.

● **Health care of adults (Chapter 8).** This covers screening in programmes for the care of persons 18 years of age and above, including the elderly. Reproductive health care issues specific to adult health care programmes are covered briefly in this chapter.

In writing the following chapters, we have relied heavily on the work of colleagues in WHO, notably in the Division of Family Health and the Division of Noncommunicable Diseases. The publications of the Canadian Task Force on the Periodic Health Examination (CTF) and the US Preventive Services Task Force (USPSTF) have been particularly helpful as source material on screening in North America. Publications from or about the United Kingdom working group on a National Child Health Surveillance Programme (UK Working Party) have also been important general sources.

CHAPTER 5

Screening in maternal, reproductive, and newborn health care

This chapter discusses screening in prenatal health care; reproductive (family) health care, which is an integral component of maternal and child health care as well as of health care for adolescents and adults; and newborn health care. Screening in the care of infants and children under 6 years of age is covered in Chapter 6 along with issues in the care of school-age children and adolescents.

Prenatal health care

General remarks[1]

Why use screening in prenatal care?

Because pregnancy is a normal condition and not a disease, a pregnant woman can be considered as asymptomatic if she is experiencing only what she considers to be the normal signs and nonpathological symptoms of pregnancy. The aim of prenatal screening is to identify the pregnant women who need surveillance and care going beyond the basic care offered to all. For example, women with certain common obstetric risk factors (e.g., a prior operative delivery or a history or risk of obstructed or prolonged labour) should be referred for care by personnel with additional training or access to facilities with more technological resources (for example, the capacity to perform an operative delivery).

Who should be screened?

Here, the emphasis is on screening procedures that should generally be performed for all pregnant women or for large subgroups, to detect risks requiring special attention. These include the screening of all pregnant women for a history of a significant disease that could affect pregnancy or the birth outcome, but not the screening indicated once a pregnant woman is diagnosed as having a given disease or pathological condition. For example, it is not within the scope of this publication to cover the testing of women with pre-existing diabetes, who require extensive pre-pregnancy as well as prenatal monitoring; of pregnant women with poor weight gain or inadequate fetal growth; or of those found to have hypertensive disease of pregnancy. Unless

---

[1] The following publications and documents were used frequently as general references for this and the following chapters and are not specifically cited every time they were used: CTF, 1979; CLAP, 1987; Hart et al., 1990; Hathaway et al., 1991; Pernoll, 1991; Program for Appropriate Technology in Health, 1984a,b; Royston & Armstrong, 1989; USPSTF, 1989; WHO/UNICEF, 1978; WHO, 1984a, 1987.

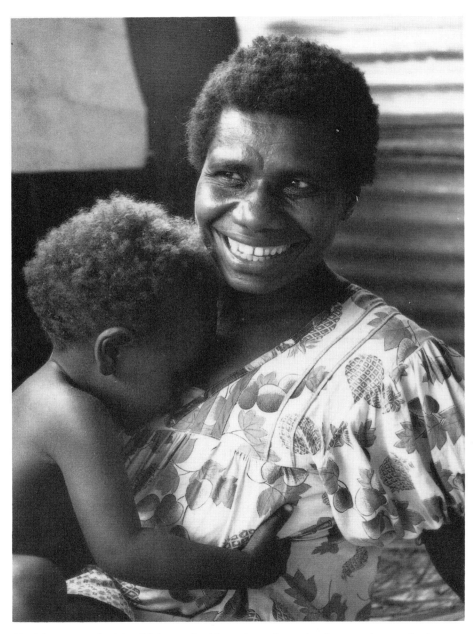

Healthy women, healthy children, a healthy society: the goals of maternal, reproductive, and child health care.   (WHO/12006)

otherwise indicated, it should be assumed that all pregnant women should be screened for the problems reviewed.

How to screen?
Screening criteria will vary with local problems and resources. For example, a report on prenatal screening for fetopelvic dystocia by auxiliary personnel in Zaire noted: "Which [choice] is selected among the reasonable [possibilities] will depend on the local circumstances: screening criteria for town women with easy access to hospital services will be different from those for a rural population living at a considerable distance. It is possible, however, even with very limited means, to provide a service which, without requiring unrealistic efforts from the population and the health services, may help to avoid a considerable number of maternal deaths" (Kasongo Project Team, 1984).

When and how frequently to screen?
There is general consensus that an initial prenatal assessment should be made in the first trimester of pregnancy. It is widely believed that care should begin as early as possible in pregnancy. Some questions have been raised about whether laboratory testing at least should be deferred until about the tenth week; many nonpreventable miscarriages will have occurred prior to that time. Some systems are experimenting with providing a promotional and educational session as soon as pregnancy is confirmed, deferring the initial screening tests until the tenth week (V. Chin, personal communication, 1993). This approach is being tested in low-risk populations with generally good access to health care services and may not be appropriate in populations with limited access, where health status is more likely to be poor, and prenatal medical risk status less well known because of poor prior access. Unless otherwise specified, all problems discussed in this section should be looked for on the first prenatal visit. Given that substantial barriers to access are widespread, except among highly affluent populations in societies with well developed national health systems, it is advisable for the first prenatal visit to be as early as possible in the pregnancy.

There is no consensus in the literature about the minimum number of prenatal screening visits for low-risk women. At least two sources suggest that, where resources are severely limited, women found on initial screening to be at no special risk should have just two prenatal screening sessions in all (one in the first trimester of pregnancy and one in the third trimester) with the emphasis on quality (Kasongo Project Team, 1984; Program for Appropriate Technology in Health, 1984a). Women found to be at special risk on the initial screening would receive additional care more frequently.

Home-based records as a screening tool

For a number of years WHO has been actively promoting the use and field-testing of simple records, kept at home, which cover the basic information needed to guide early detection and health promotion activities in the area of

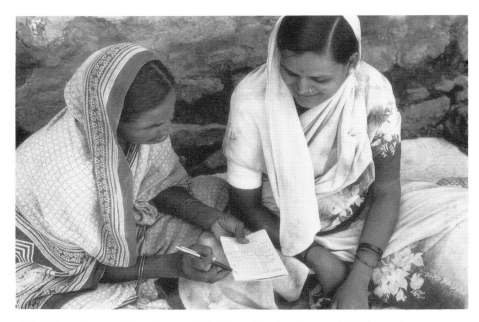

A health worker explains the use of the home-based mother and child record.

maternal and child health (WHO, 1994). Originally developed in rural India in the 1970s, the "home-based mother's card" appears to be a useful tool for the primary health care worker and to guide screening.

A record of the basic obstetric history for up to three pregnancies and the intervals between them can be kept on one card. The health worker is supplied with blank cards by the health post or centre. The health worker keeps either a logbook or a duplicate of each card on thin paper, while the original multipanel card, on thick paper and protected by a plastic covering, is kept by the woman concerned. The cards guide prenatal and postpartum screening by specifying essential information to be recorded by tick marks, using simple language or pictorial symbols appropriate to the local culture where the literacy of health workers may be limited. They record such essential data as: reproductive complications and outcomes (e.g., obstructed labour, a low-birth-weight baby, or a stillbirth), complications during pregnancy and delivery (e.g., excessive oedema or increased blood pressure), immunization status, and general medical risks such as a history of tuberculosis.

The home-based record appears to be an extremely useful means of educating mothers as well as traditional birth attendants and other community health workers, and of providing guidance on the content and timetable of early detection, screening, and health promotion activities. Another function is to document the risks detected by screening at the primary care level in a way that facilitates the process of referral between the community or peripheral post, the health centre, and the district hospital (Shah & Shah, 1981; Shah et al., 1988; WHO, 1994). Experience to date indicates very high rates of

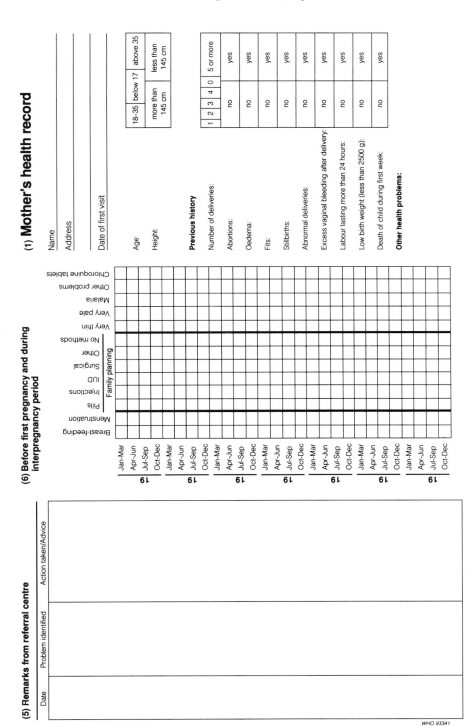

(1) Mother's health record

Name

Address

Date of first visit

	18–35	below 17	above 35
Age:			
Height:	more than 145 cm		less than 145 cm

Previous history

Number of deliveries:	1	2	3	4	0	5 or more
Abortions:	no					yes
Oedema:	no					yes
Fits:	no					yes
Stillbirths:	no					yes
Abnormal deliveries:	no					yes
Excess vaginal bleeding after delivery:	no					yes
Labour lasting more than 24 hours:	no					yes
Low birth weight (less than 2500 g):	no					yes
Death of child during first week:	no					yes

Other health problems:

(6) Before first pregnancy and during interpregnancy period

(5) Remarks from referral centre

Date	Problem identified	Action taken/Advice

WHO 93341

The WHO prototype home-based maternal record, parts 1, 5 and 6

53

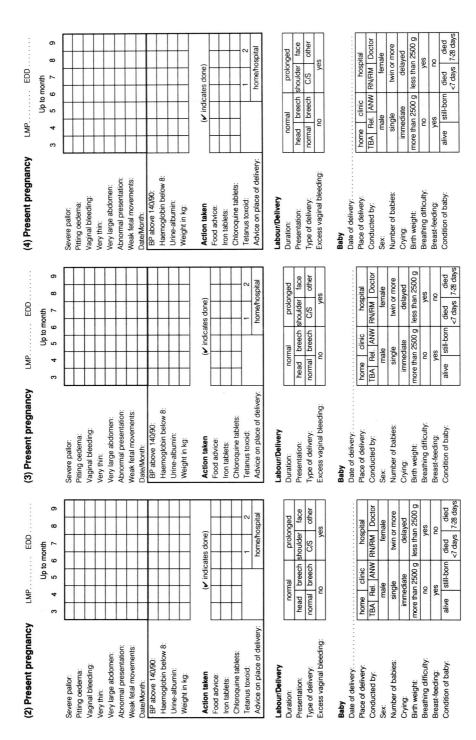

The WHO prototype home-based maternal record, parts 2, 3 and 4

compliance in keeping the home-based records on hand at home and bringing them to health care visits.

Health education

Outreach and mass public education, targeting but not restricted to women, may also be required to ensure that all pregnant women seek care as early as possible in pregnancy. Public education may also be important to ensure that the health needs of pregnant women including nutritional and other needs detected on screening and the need for health services are given priority within the family and the community. These issues were discussed in Chapter 3.

Prenatal screening in primary health care

● **Prior complication of pregnancy, labour or delivery,** including premature or prolonged labour, haemorrhage, caesarean section, hypertensive disease of pregnancy (as manifested by severe oedema or convulsions); or prior adverse pregnancy outcome (miscarriage, stillbirth, low birth weight, or premature birth) (Kasongo Project Team, 1984; Program for Appropriate Technology in Health, 1984a).

Why. To identify women at high risk of complications in a current pregnancy, in order to refer them for care by personnel or centres suitably equipped to prevent maternal and neonatal morbidity and mortality. An adverse obstetric history is an excellent indicator of risk in a current pregnancy.

How and when. By enquiry or inspection of home-based records at initial prenatal visit; this may be done by trained auxiliary health workers. A study from Zaire, in which auxiliary personnel were trained to screen women for fetopelvic disproportion, concluded that a history of prolonged labour in a previous pregnancy or of a stillbirth or early neonatal loss was the most cost-effective indicator of a life-threatening fetopelvic disproportion. Other indicators looked at in the same study included very short stature, parity (no or one prior birth), and age. Indicators other than obstetric history needed to be combined to produce an adequate predictive value (Kasongo Project Team, 1984).

Resource levels required. Low for detection by enquiry or inspection of home-based records. Medium or high for definitive diagnosis and intervention (referral to a centre with more trained personnel and a capacity for operative delivery).

Recommendation on use of screening. Recommended. Although a medium or high level of resources is required for intervention, such resources should be a basic component of any district's health services. Early intervention is of proven effectiveness in preventing maternal mortality and serious neonatal morbidity and mortality.

● **Age or parity indicating high risk**

Why. To identify women who should be referred to a centre with the capacity for operative delivery, because of risks associated with extremes of age or parity.

How and when. Through enquiry and/or history at initial prenatal visit; may be carried out by trained auxiliary health workers. Criteria for high risk vary widely; for example, age over 35 (or over 30 and primiparous) or under 15 (17 in some areas), or any age with 5 or more previous births are commonly used criteria. Younger women (under 18 or under 16) with no or only one prior birth may be at increased risk of fetopelvic disproportion, especially if short in stature or if abdominal examination in the third trimester reveals failure of the head to engage; however, an adverse obstetric history is in itself a better indicator of risk. The threshold for referral to more highly trained staff or for additional local surveillance alone will vary according to the constraints on access to referral facilities.

Resource levels required. Low for detection; medium or high for timely intervention.

Recommendation on use of screening. Recommended. Although a medium or high level of resources is required for intervention, such resources should be a basic component of any district's health services. Early intervention is of proven effectiveness in preventing maternal mortality and serious neonatal morbidity and mortality.

● **Short stature**

Why. Very short women are at high risk of fetopelvic disproportion and need to be referred to a centre with the capacity for operative delivery, especially as the time for delivery approaches.

How and when. By inspection at the first prenatal visit. Assess height using, for example, a string calibrated according to appropriate population criteria. Can be done by primary care workers.

Where. Can be done wherever a means of measurement is available, e.g., at the women's home if a calibrated string is brought by the health worker, or at a health post using markings on a wall.

Resource levels required. Low for detection; medium (pelvic examination) or high (X-ray pelvimetry) for diagnosis; medium or high for intervention (obstetric provider with ability to perform instrumentally assisted or operative delivery, if obstructed labour occurs).

Recommendation on use of screening. Recommended. Operative delivery (caesarean section or assisted vaginal delivery) in women with fetopelvic disproportion can prevent maternal and fetal death and major morbidity. A capacity for assisted and operative delivery is an essential component of any district health care system.

● **Maternal immunization status** (tetanus, rubella)

Why. To immunize those who have not completed the basic course of antitetanus injections or who need an antitetanus booster; to advise those not immunized against rubella on precautions against exposure and to arrange for postpartum immunization to prevent congenital rubella syndrome in a subsequent pregnancy.

How and when. Through enquiry or review of home-based or clinical records at the initial prenatal visit. Tetanus immunization should be given when immunization status is in doubt and records are inadequate. Ideally, rubella antibody titres should be checked if status is uncertain; otherwise, immunize postpartum if any doubt.

Resource levels required. Low for detection (enquiry or inspection of records); medium for measuring rubella antibody titre; low for intervention (immunization).

Recommendation on use of screening. Recommended. Screening is of low cost and high effectiveness in preventing neonatal tetanus and congenital rubella syndrome.

● **Psychosocial and socioeconomic risks in the household**

Why. Common important psychosocial risks include: inadequate social support; domestic violence or history of child abuse or neglect; abuse of alcohol or other substances in the household. Unemployment of household members counted on as wage-earners, or a precarious financial situation, puts pregnant women and the household at risk and can precipitate or exacerbate psychosocial risks. Such risks might be assessed by observation and enquiry regarding special problems throughout the prenatal and postnatal period. The objective of early detection of these factors is to provide additional surveillance and support by the health worker and referral to other community resources (e.g., women's groups, social services, church groups) where they exist. Early detection of psychosocial and socioeconomic risks among pregnant women could not only identify the pregnant woman or child that will be at risk; it could also identify the at-risk household whose members require help.

How and when. Through history and observation by a worker trained in detection and in the rudiments of supportive counselling or referral. Risk factors that apply to other family members, especially children, should be noted. Family records are of help in carrying over information on risk factors; the best way of ensuring this is to have a system of services that is strong at the primary care level, with primary care workers who know their community. As a minimum, such workers can routinely ask all pregnant women whether they are under any particular stress at home or at work for which they need help, or which they would like to discuss.

Resource levels required. Low or medium for initial detection, depending in part on the nature and complexity of the problem; uncertain level needed for definitive diagnosis and intervention. Intervention at a low or medium level (e.g., social support, supportive counselling) may be effective for certain problems.

Recommendation on use of screening/early detection. This set of conditions fits an "early detection" model rather than "screening" as strictly interpreted. Early detection is recommended as an adjunct to primary prevention. Psychosocial and economic assistance through community networks should be available for those found to be at elevated risk. Assessment of psychosocial and socioeconomic risk should be a standard component of prenatal screening in many health care delivery systems, especially for low-income populations.

Research priority. To develop valid low-cost primary care and community-based methods of assessing and dealing with psychosocial and socioeconomic risks in the prenatal period. The primary prevention of social and economic risks through a humane social policy is essential and far more important than screening, and should be given the highest priority in a preventive strategy.

● Barriers to access (subsequent receipt of health care services)

Why. In order to target pregnant women with poor access to services for special outreach and promotional efforts. The problem of access may be financial (cost of visit, prescribed medicines, or transport), linguistic, geographical, or related to problems of child care or economic responsibilities that interfere with obtaining care; or it may be related to lack of knowledge or to negative perceptions of health services or care providers.

Outreach and broad public education should always be performed, along with measures to reduce logistic barriers to health care, in the population as a whole. In addition, effort should be focused on identifying those who have made an initial visit for prenatal care but who are at risk of not returning for recommended care, who may be helped by simple supportive measures.

How and when. Enquiry at initial visit regarding means of transport, travel time, and problems getting to health care services. Review of home-based or clinical records may also help identify women with barriers to access (under-utilization in the past).

Resource levels required. Low for detection. Intervention may be at a low resource level, for example, providing special support through home visits, helping with child care or transport for visits, or providing a translator.

Recommendation on use of screening. Recommended as an adjunct to primary prevention. Early identification of barriers to access among those already using services is only an adjunct to the universal promotion of financial and geographical access and measures dealing with other barriers to utilization of needed care.

● **Smoking and use of alcohol or other harmful substances by expectant mothers**

Why. To counsel and offer support for stopping use of harmful substances.

How and when. Enquiry and review of records at initial prenatal visit. Assurance of confidentiality must be given and respected; fear of legal repercussions (e.g., loss of custody of child or other punitive measures) will reduce chances of detection.

Resource levels required. Low for detection; low, medium, or high for intervention, i.e., counselling and support for the mother, and special surveillance, medical, and psychosocial treatment for infants of drug-dependent mothers.

Recommendation on use of screening/early detection. Early detection recommended only as an adjunct to primary prevention. During pregnancy, a woman's motivation to make difficult changes in behaviour is often relatively high, and some studies have shown that counselling by a trusted health care provider can help. Appropriate support for cessation of substance use should be offered to any woman requiring it, for the sake of the health of the woman, her unborn child and the rest of her family. Additional social support can be offered and note taken of vulnerable households and unborn children who should receive additional surveillance and support after birth to reduce the risk of neglect or abuse. Arrangements to screen pregnant women for problems of substance use can be only a minor adjunct to an effective policy for the prevention of such problems, which depends on broad social measures.

Research priority. Low-cost community-based methods of counselling for stopping substance use during pregnancy.

● **Poor nutritional status, weight gain, or fetal growth**

Why. To prevent low birth weight and maternal morbidity by counselling and education aimed at promoting optimal nutritional intake (including family counselling to ensure that the needs of the pregnant woman have priority); by giving supplements when available; by referring women to a birth facility equipped to care for low-birth-weight babies.

How. A dietary history may be helpful. Ideally, assess by weight, if scales are available, and check fundal height with a tape measure (Mathai, 1988;

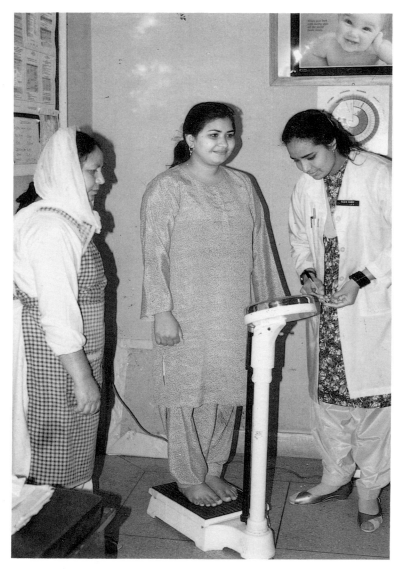

Weight monitoring in prenatal screening: equipment such as scales requires not only an initial purchase but careful maintenance.

WHO, 1986b). If scales are not available, it may be possible to train workers to assess by inspection the weight status of women whose initial weight is grossly under or above the normal range, but it will be impossible to follow weight gain during pregnancy in this way.

When. Assess general nutritional status at the initial visit and weight gain/status at each routine visit.

Resource levels required. Low (scales for weight gain; measuring-tape for fundal height) for screening; low, medium (laboratory tests) or high (ultrasound) for definitive diagnosis; low, medium, or high for intervention.

Recommendation on use of screening. Recommended only when adequate supplementation and effective counselling are available for women at risk. Primary prevention should have highest priority. Screening may be useful where adequate supplementation is available for all those found to have a poor overall nutritional status. However, where nutritional inadequacies are widespread and supplementation is limited, nutritional counselling is of unproven effectiveness among women with problems. A more rational strategy would be to improve food supply on a community-wide basis, and generally promote good nutritional status and education about the extra needs of pregnant and lactating women. General promotion of the status of women will also be important in societies with limited food supplies where women are sometimes given the lowest priority for the available food. (**Note:** Routine ultrasound for gestational age determination to assess fetal growth is **not** recommended.)

● **Occupational risks,** e.g., woman performs heavy manual labour or is exposed to potential teratogens at work.

Why. Heavy manual work is a risk factor for premature labour (Program for Appropriate Technology in Health, 1984a). The reason for screening would presumably be to counsel women to avoid heavy manual labour or exposure to potential teratogens. However, there is no evidence that counselling by health providers is effective when the household's economic situation depends on the woman's labour, and in the absence of appropriate regulations and laws governing working conditions.

How and when. By enquiry at initial prenatal visit.

Resource levels required. Low for detection, variable for definitive diagnosis; intervention requires cessation of activities that put mother at risk, or removal of source of risk from the workplace.

Recommendation on use of screening. Uncertain. Especially where there is a very low-income population dependent on the earnings of every family member, the effectiveness of counselling women on the health risks of exposures at work is uncertain. Primary prevention through policies promoting safe working conditions for all and social recognition of the special needs of pregnant women are essential.

● **History of chronic disease or neglected acute/recent symptoms:** a history of chronic disease (e.g., tuberculosis, hepatitis, asthma, hypertension, diabetes, heart disease, or a debilitating mental health problem) (Program for

Appropriate Technology in Health, 1984a); or a history of recent neglected symptoms suggesting acute illness that requires medical care (e.g., fever in a malaria-endemic area; malaria is a major contributory factor to perinatal mortality in some areas (Program for Appropriate Technology in Health, 1984a; WHO, 1989a)); symptoms of genitourinary infection (e.g., discharge, dysuria) or a history of exposure to sexually transmitted disease.

Why. To ensure appropriate treatment to prevent maternal and neonatal morbidity and mortality.

How and when. By enquiry or review of records at initial prenatal visit.

Resource levels required. Low or medium for detection (the detection of certain conditions may require trained personnel); medium or high for definitive diagnosis; low, medium, or high for appropriate timely intervention, depending on the condition.

Recommendation on use of screening/early detection. Early detection is recommended as an adjunct to primary prevention. The basic services within a district health system should be capable of detecting and treating the most common chronic conditions that are treatable without extremely expensive resources and that could compromise maternal, fetal or neonatal health. The entire population should be educated to practise self-referral for symptoms, and women with chronic disease should be under special surveillance or promotional care.

● Iron deficiency anaemia

Why. To give dietary supplements and advice, or refer for treatment for other causes, e.g., malaria or other parasitic or bacterial infections. Anaemia, even moderate, is associated with adverse birth outcome, including premature delivery, and with maternal morbidity; it may be asymptomatic especially where health status generally is poor.

How and when. By blood test at initial visit. The Talqvist technique for estimating haemoglobin appears more appropriate than the copper sulfate method (Program for Appropriate Technology in Health, 1984a; WHO, 1984a). It has been suggested that, where basic laboratory facilities are lacking, it may be possible to train workers to look for clinical signs of anaemia and refer those showing them for definitive diagnosis; the value of this approach has not been confirmed, and it falls into the category of early detection rather than screening.

Resource levels required. Low or medium for initial screening; low (response to iron) or medium (laboratory tests, including complete blood count with indices) for definitive diagnosis; iron studies or haemoglobin electrophoresis may be indicated later but are not likely to be essential as part of initial work-up; low for intervention (iron or dietary supplementation).

Recommendation on use of screening. Recommended. Screening accompanied by supplementation and dietary counselling should not take the place of primary prevention efforts through the community-wide promotion of better nutritional status for the entire population. If screening with validated blood-testing cannot be provided to the entire population, with priority for those at greatest risk of iron deficiency (lowest socioeconomic groups, teenagers, older or high-parity women), then early detection of those showing clinical signs is preferable to screening only the relatively privileged groups.

● Malaria

Why. Malaria is an important cause of maternal and perinatal mortality in endemic areas, may have asymptomatic phases, and is treatable. Infection in pregnancy can cause intrauterine growth retardation or premature delivery; it is unlikely to result in fetal infection.

Who. All pregnant women in endemic areas.

How and when. Through blood smear on first prenatal visit, according to local testing protocols.

Resource levels required. Low or medium for detection (laboratory examination of blood smear according to local protocols); low or medium for intervention (chloroquine or other medication).

Recommendation on use of screening. Recommended in endemic areas as an adjunct to primary prevention, which should have the highest priority. Primary prevention would reduce malarial infection through environmental measures and public education, eliminating sites where the mosquito vector breeds and reducing human and animal exposure to mosquito bites. Effective intervention generally requires household or community-level environmental action to prevent reinfection.

● Iodine deficiency

Why. Congenital hypothyroidism due to iodine deficiency, if untreated, leads to irreversible damage to the central nervous system; iodine supplementation within the first 1–2 months of life can prevent this.

Who. Pregnant women living in areas where iodine deficiency is common.

How. Accurate, reliable detection in pregnancy is difficult; urine assays require 24-hour collection, which is often impractical, and most blood tests for triiodothyronine (T_3), thyroxine (T_4), and thyroid-stimulating hormone (TSH) are expensive; screening of newborns in endemic areas by testing samples of cord blood is less expensive and intervention is effective if initiated within the first 2 months of life (Program for Appropriate Technology in Health, 1987) (see page 81).

Resource levels required. High for urine/blood assays in pregnant women; cord-blood assay in newborns is less expensive; low for intervention (iodine supplementation).

Recommendation on use of screening. Prenatal screening not recommended. Primary prevention through universal iodine supplementation in endemic areas is most rational, combined with neonatal screening and early detection of palpable goitres in pregnant women.

● Multiple gestation, breech or transverse lie

Why. Multiple gestation and malposition both indicate the need for more intensive support to prevent maternal or neonatal morbidity and mortality, and risk of need for operative delivery.

How and when. Initial screening by pelvic examination during third trimester of pregnancy. Hygienic facilities for pelvic examination should be one of the highest priorities in developing local health services. However, if these cannot be provided, abdominal examination at least should be performed to try to detect possible multiple gestation or breech position.

Resource levels required. Detection: low for abdominal examination; medium for pelvic examination; high for definitive diagnosis with ultrasound, but this may not be essential if the examiner is highly skilled. Intervention: medium for forceps delivery (vacuum extraction may involve a high or medium level of resources); high for caesarean section.

Recommendation on use of screening. Recommended. Timely intervention to deal with a malpositioned fetus will prevent maternal and fetal morbidity and mortality; primary care workers should be able to perform screening in places far away from any hospital. Fetal prospects may be improved if multiple gestation is detected early and the mother is referred to a centre with the capacity for operative delivery.

● Hypertensive disease of pregnancy (pre-eclampsia, eclampsia, toxaemia of pregnancy)

Why. This is a major treatable cause of maternal and fetal morbidity and mortality. Can be treated with bed rest, magnesium sulfate, or induction of labour; operative delivery may be necessary.

How. Assess by measuring blood pressure, as well as performing physical examination for oedema of face or hands or excessive oedema of lower extremities (early detection). Also check urine for protein, using a dipstick, if available; low-cost dipsticks have been developed, and there are alternative low-cost laboratory methods (Program for Appropriate Technology

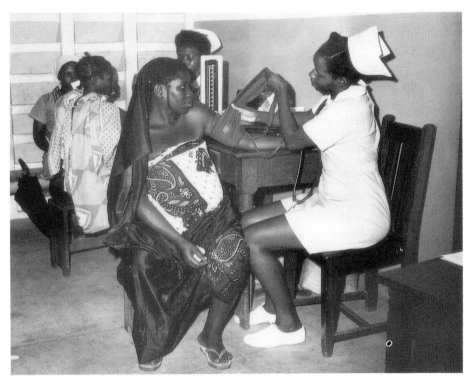

Checking blood pressure as part of prenatal care in the United Republic of Tanzania.
(P. Almasy/WHO/20924)

in Health, 1984a). If a blood pressure cuff is unavailable, an assessment can be made by enquiring about symptoms and examining for physical signs; this would be an example of early detection rather than screening.

When. At each visit.

Resource levels required. Low for detection (blood pressure cuff, physical examination, urine reagent strips); low (bed rest), medium, or high for intervention (medication, induction of labour, or operative delivery in severe cases).

Recommendation on use of screening. Recommended. Detection is easy; the condition is a common cause of maternal and fetal morbidity and mortality; intervention is effective and should be an essential part of district health services.

● Asymptomatic bacteriuria

Why. Asymptomatic urinary tract infection in pregnancy is associated with premature labour and subsequent symptomatic infection in the mother; these can be prevented with antibiotic treatment.

How and when*.* Assessment on initial visit, by microscopic examination of urine for pyuria or bacteriuria. Chemical dipsticks are available for the detection of white cells (by identifying leukocyte esterase) or bacteriuria (by nitrite reduction, which has lower sensitivity but better specificity than leukocyte esterase screening tests). (The US Preventive Services Task Force has data on the sensitivity, specificity, and predictive value of different screening methods for asymptomatic bacteriuria in pregnant women and others.) Pyuria may indicate infection with *Neisseria gonorrhoeae* or *Chlamydia trachomatis* (see below). The expense of dipstick tests may be greater than that of microscopic examination, if enough trained personnel are available for the latter. Urine culture is more sensitive and specific, but also more expensive, and requires at least 24 hours for results, which may be impractical in many places with populations that are difficult to reach.

Resource levels required*.* Low (dipsticks for urine) or medium (urinalysis by trained personnel) for screening; medium (urine culture) for definitive diagnosis unless a urological work-up is required for repeated infections/ treatment failures; low or medium (antibiotics) for intervention.

Recommendation on use of screening*.* Recommended. Detection and intervention are relatively inexpensive and easy to do; intervention is of proven effectiveness in preventing premature labour. Primary prevention through education of girls and women about perineal hygiene is also needed.

● Infection with *Neisseria gonorrhoeae*, *Chlamydia trachomatis*, and other common sexually transmitted copathogens

Why*.* To prevent neonatal ophthalmia (*N. gonorrhoeae*) and pneumonitis (*C. trachomatis*) and maternal morbidity (pelvic inflammatory disease with potential sequela of permanent infertility). These sexually transmitted diseases are often asymptomatic; mixed infections are common.

How and when*.* Assessment on initial visit by culture for *N. gonorrhoeae* from the cervix or urethra. Pelvic examination can be performed in a health post with basic equipment and supplies. Timely access to a microbiology laboratory is also needed. In many areas *C. trachomatis* is more prevalent and appears to be associated with more severe morbidity than *N. gonorrhoeae*. Screening tests for *Chlamydia* were relatively expensive in the past, but less costly methods have been developed recently. Decisions about screening for *Chlamydia* would depend on local prevalence or incidence and resources. In the United States, the current protocol in areas of significant prevalence is to treat presumptively for chlamydial infection if the gonorrhoea test is positive or if pelvic examination reveals mucopurulent cervicitis.

Resource levels required*.* Low or medium for screening (urine dipstick for pyuria; abnormal vaginal/cervical discharge or cervical inflammation noted on visual examination); medium or high (culture) for definitive diagnosis, which may not be essential; low or medium for intervention (antibiotics).

Recommendation on use of screening. Recommended. Resources needed for testing and treating pregnant women for asymptomatic gonorrhoea are relatively low and such testing should be part of local health services. Intervention is of proven effectiveness in preventing serious maternal and neonatal morbidity. Screening is an adjunct to primary prevention through community-wide promotion of safe sexual practices.

• Syphilis

Why. Congenital syphilis is preventable with antibiotic treatment during pregnancy. If untreated, it is associated with a high risk of fetal or perinatal death, serious complications in surviving newborns, and permanent neurological or cardiovascular sequelae in the mothers (Bhat et al., 1982; Stray-Pedersen, 1983).

How and when. By serum VDRL (Venereal Disease Research Laboratory) test on initial prenatal visit.

Resource levels required. Medium or high technology but low cost for screening (VDRL); medium or high technology but low cost for definitive diagnosis (rapid plasma reagin test); medium for treatment (antibiotics, possibly parenteral).

Recommendation on use of screening. Recommended. Prenatal testing for syphilis should be a high priority. Testing requires a blood sample and laboratory facilities (medium or high technological level; may require central laboratory but testing is inexpensive in high numbers); treatment requires trained personnel (medium level) but cost is low. Screening is an adjunct to primary prevention through community-wide promotion of safe sexual practices.

• HIV infection in pregnancy

Why. Voluntary testing of asymptomatic individuals may be a useful adjunct to primary prevention (education and condom distribution), especially to allow care and support to be given to infected individuals. It has not been demonstrated to reduce the risk of further transmission, however. Involuntary testing, testing without informed consent, and testing without appropriate pre- and post-test counselling are unethical and ineffective. A negative test result may give a false sense of security, so that the person may continue to indulge in behaviour that puts her at risk. Zidovudine therapy appears to prolong survival and quality of life for symptomatic persons with HIV infection, but early treatment of asymptomatic HIV-infected persons may not be beneficial (Anon., 1993). The extremely high expense of such therapy means that it is not a realistic option for most developing countries.

Who. Pregnant women who are at elevated risk and who have given informed consent. Women can be considered at elevated risk if they or their partner: has a number of sexual partners; has a sexually transmitted disease; uses illicit injectable drugs; or has received injections in unhygienic conditions; or if their partner is bisexual.

How and when. Testing should be confidential and voluntary, with informed consent and pre- and post-test counselling. Blood tests are available that give results within hours and are relatively reliable in high-risk populations; there will be a high false-positive rate in low-risk populations. Voluntary prenatal testing for HIV infection should be done as early in pregnancy as possible but only after adequate pre-test counselling. Pre- and post-test counselling requires highly trained and skilled health workers.

Resource levels required. Medium or high for detection, including skilled pre-test counselling; medium or high for skilled post-test counselling on whether to continue pregnancy, on breast-feeding, and on ways of prolonging the symptom-free state. A range of resource levels (from low to very high) is possible for interventions to promote quality of life and survival in HIV-positive individuals, including social support and other supportive services at the primary care level.

Recommendation on use of screening. Uncertain. Universal confidential voluntary screening of pregnant women in high-prevalence areas may allow infected women to choose therapeutic abortion, make an informed decision on breast-feeding, or receive appropriate care. However, skilled pre- and post-test counselling must be available in order to make testing an effective use of resources. Screening should not be used as a substitute for primary prevention, through community-wide education on safe sexual practices, making condoms readily available, and preventing parenteral transmission (contaminated needles); these approaches must have first priority in a preventive strategy.

In many developing countries, parenteral transmission is not only an issue for professional medical and dental care providers and for users of illicit intravenous drugs. Injections are often given by family members or relatively untrained lay personnel in the community working outside the formal health services, and education must reach these informal care providers as well. Treatment programmes need to be available for intravenous drug abusers; motivation to stop using drugs is often high during pregnancy. Programmes providing clean needles or disinfectants (chlorine bleach) to drug users are controversial but appear to have been associated with reductions in the rate of new HIV infections (see page 113).

● Hepatitis B infection

Why. Hepatitis B infection is one of the principal etiological factors for primary liver cancer throughout the world. Primary liver cancer is among the major causes of death from cancer in a number of developing countries, especially in Asia and, to a lesser extent, in Africa. Where vaccination of newborn infants against hepatitis B is not universal, the testing of pregnant women for hepatitis B surface antigen (HBsAg) allows newborn babies of infected mothers to be vaccinated and thus protected against chronic hepatitis and primary liver cancer in adult life (Sun et al., 1986; Arevalo & Washington, 1988).

How and when. Blood test at the first prenatal visit.

Resource levels required. Medium (testing for HBsAg) or high (testing for infectivity) for detection; medium or high for administering hepatitis vaccine (3 separate doses) and hepatitis immune globulin to newborns of antigen-positive mothers.

Recommendation on use of screening. Recommended as a priority only in communities with vertical transmission (i.e., from mother to fetus) and an HBsAg prevalence of under 10%. Before investing in this strategy, preliminary studies are required to establish that vertical transmission is an important mode of spread (Shrestha, 1987). In communities where the prevalence is 10% or more, the universal vaccination of all newborns may be more efficient and effective than screening; screening would not be recommended in such circumstances. Primary prevention through promotion of safe sexual practices and the prevention of intravenous drug abuse is also important.

• ABO blood group

Why. In case of maternal blood loss requiring transfusion.

How and when. Blood test at initial visit.

Resource levels required. Medium or high for detection (testing at central laboratory); high for intervention (transfusion).

Recommendation on use of screening. Recommended. Where resources are too limited for the entire population to be tested, first priority should go to those women most likely to require operative delivery, or those with a history of intrapartum or postpartum haemorrhage.

• Rhesus (Rh) antibodies

Why. To give Rh immune globulin to the Rh-negative mother of a Rh-positive baby or fetus so as to prevent life-threatening haemolytic anaemia in a subsequent child, in case isoimmunization has occurred during pregnancy or delivery.

How and when. Blood test at initial visit.

Resource levels required. Medium or high for detection (central laboratory); high for treatment (Rh immune globulin to Rh-negative mother after delivery of Rh-positive baby).

Recommendation on use of screening. Recommended, but of lower priority than for the conditions listed above. Detection and intervention for the more common of these conditions should have first priority where resources are particularly limited.

● Gestational diabetes

Why. Screening has been performed to detect gestational diabetes in order to intervene with diet or insulin to prevent macrosomia and other complications.

How, when, and resource levels required. There is no simple, non-invasive, inexpensive screening test for gestational diabetes that is sufficiently accurate. Accurate diagnosis requires a 50-g oral glucose tolerance test (administration of glucose load followed by timed serial measurements of blood sugar) at 24–28 weeks of gestation (USPSTF, 1989). Detection requires a medium level of technology but is expensive because of the need for repeated serial measurements. Intervention requires low (if dietary counselling is adequate) to medium (insulin) resource levels.

Recommendation on use of screening. Not recommended as a priority. While gestational diabetes is a risk factor for macrosomia, which increases the risk of birth trauma to child and mother, obesity is a far more important risk factor (USPSTF, 1989; Al-Shawaf et al., 1988; Ng et al., 1981). Pregnant women with pre-existing (juvenile-onset-type) diabetes mellitus account for a very small proportion of pregnant women, should already be known by prior history, and should be under special care. There is no reliable evidence of an association between gestational diabetes and the more serious adverse effects associated with juvenile-onset diabetes (Braveman et al., 1988). Within a primary health care system, the allocation of resources to counselling and support aimed at reducing obesity would be more rational than routine testing for gestational diabetes. Where some resources are available for testing for gestational diabetes, it would be rational to give priority to obese women and to those with a history of a macrosomic infant, followed by older women of higher parity.

● Routine prenatal/intrapartum electronic fetal monitoring for fetal asphyxia

Recommendation on use of screening. Not recommended as a priority in the case of low-risk pregnancies. Detection and intervention are very expensive and of uncertain effectiveness. There is controversy regarding possible adverse consequences of the routine use of electronic fetal monitoring for low-risk pregnancies. Fetal heart rate should be monitored "by auscultation on all women in labour to detect signs of fetal distress. Electronic fetal monitoring ... should be reserved for pregnancies at increased risk of fetal distress" (USPSTF, 1989).

● Prenatal genetic screening

Prenatal genetic screening includes screening for chromosomal abnormalities associated with serious birth defects, screening for direct evidence of congenital structural anomalies, and screening for haemoglobinopathies and other inherited conditions detectable by biochemical assay. Universal genetic screening is generally not recommended as a priority within a primary health care strategy, because of the very high resource levels required for screening, diagnosis, and effective preventive action, and the alternative strategies for primary prevention that might be a better use of resources. Highly skilled counselling services are an essential component of the screening as well as of the preventive action that goes with it; considerable professional training and expense are involved in both the counselling and the testing. A rational strategy will emphasize primary prevention through informed family planning, reduction of exposure to teratogens, and improved maternal nutrition.

● Screening for chromosomal abnormalities associated with severe birth defects, and screening by ultrasound for direct evidence of structural anomalies

Why. Screening for chromosomal abnormalities and for direct evidence of structural anomalies is performed in pregnancy in order to make the option of therapeutic abortion available when severe defects are detected. Typical examples are screening for trisomy 21 (Down syndrome) and severe neural tube defects; the possibility of serum screening for other serious chromosomal abnormalities is currently being studied (Modell et al., 1991).

Who. Women aged 35 years and above and those who already have an afflicted child are at higher risk, but to use such criteria for screening would mean missing many cases. The costs of karyotyping all women would be prohibitive and the risk:benefit ratio unacceptably high. Multistage screening methods have been used to screen all women initially, using serum assays, age criteria, and sometimes ultrasound to establish a high-risk subgroup for karyotyping (see below).

How and when. Karyotyping for chromosomal abnormalities can be done via amniocentesis (usually in the second trimester) or the newer method of chorionic villus sampling (CVS) (in the first trimester). The most efficient method of screening for the detection of Down syndrome is a multistage one: serum assays of maternal alphafetoprotein, combined with other maternal biochemical assays in the second trimester, are interpreted in the light of maternal age to establish a subgroup of women at particularly high risk who should then receive karyotyping by amniocentesis or CVS (Modell et al., 1991). If serum screening in the first trimester were to become available, this would make it possible to perform CVS (and, if indicated and desired, therapeutic abortion) earlier, which would have distinct psychological advantages for the patients. Karyotyping is far more expensive than serum assay and carries certain risks (spontaneous abortion, infection, and bleeding). In some developed countries with high rates of neural tube defects, ultrasonography has been considered for the routine screening of all pregnant women. It must, however, be combined with serum alphafetoprotein assays to have an acceptable degree of sensitivity. Rigorous assessments of evidence on the safety and clinical efficacy of routine ultrasound screening in pregnancy have not reached any definitive conclusions (USPSTF, 1989; Modell et al., 1991).

Resource levels required. High or very high for screening, including skilled pre- and post-test counselling; very high for diagnosis. Therapeutic abortion requires only a medium level of resources. However, specialized resources are necessary for the difficult counselling required for those who test positive (Grace, 1981; USPSTF, 1989). Modell et al. (1991) recommend that qualified midwives or other "appropriate primary care workers" should be trained to perform the counselling required for genetic services in Europe, in order to improve continuity of care and ensure a more sensitive approach.

Recommendation on use of screening. Not recommended as a priority. Recommended alternatives include an emphasis on primary prevention by decreasing toxic exposures (including to alcohol and occupational and environmental mutagens), providing safe, accessible, and acceptable family planning services, and discouraging pregnancy in women aged 35 and over and in those who have already had afflicted children (Henderson, 1982; PAHO, 1984; USPSTF, 1989). According to a recent WHO publication (Modell et al., 1991), "Family planning alone seems to have reduced the incidence of Down's syndrome in Europe by between 30% and 60%, depending on the country." Congenital rubella syndrome can be prevented by immunization. Recent evidence suggests that adequate maternal intake of folate can prevent neural tube defects. Health systems that can ensure universal access to services that are able to carry out second-trimester alphafetoprotein screening, along with adequate counselling and follow-up, may want to introduce such screening.

● **Haemoglobinopathies** and other inherited diseases that may be detected prenatally through biochemical assays

Why. Prenatal screening for inherited conditions, through biochemical assays, is performed to detect fetal conditions associated with mortality or serious disabling morbidity, such as thalassaemia major, cystic fibrosis, Duchenne muscular dystrophy, Huntington chorea, haemophilia A and B, and alpha-1 antitrypsin deficiency). The purpose of such testing is to give women the option of therapeutic abortion. The effectiveness of counselling regarding future pregnancy risks (as opposed to conditions present in the current pregnancy) is not known.

How and when. Biochemical assays are now available for the prenatal detection of many inherited diseases. Such screening should be offered as early as possible in pregnancy.

Resource levels required. Medium for tests for sickle-cell haemoglobin; high for detection of other haemoglobinopathies and other inherited diseases. Pre- and post-test genetic counselling requires highly specialized training.

Recommendation on use of screening. Not recommended as a priority in view of the expense of testing and counselling. The impact on current and future pregnancies of counselling following prenatal screening should be studied locally before resources are invested in such a programme. Neonatal (rather than prenatal) screening for sickle-cell disease (homozygous condition) is recommended in areas of high prevalence (see page 83). Where an adequate infrastructure exists, screening targeted to particularly high-risk groups may be worth while.

Reproductive (family) health care

Reproductive or "family" health care should be seen as an integral component of prenatal and postpartum care, as well as of care in the interpregnancy period. It should also be integrated into programmes for well-baby and well-child care and health care programmes for adolescents and adults. Generally, outside maternal and child health care, the screening relevant to reproductive health care is "opportunistic", i.e., it is performed as opportunities arise when persons seek health services for other reasons. The one exception is screening for cancer of the uterine cervix, which women should be taught to seek at appropriate intervals as an essential part of their routine health care.

In prenatal and postpartum care, the home-based mother's record provides a useful tool to guide screening for reproductive health risks (e.g., high parity, short interpregnancy interval, adverse pregnancy outcome), and can serve as a reminder to health care providers to address family planning issues (Shah et al., 1988). Reproductive health care should also be integrated into routine health care for adolescents in schools and neighbourhoods and for adults at their places of work and in other community and institutional settings.

● Risk of unintended or high-risk pregnancy in the future

Why. In order to provide education/counselling and, when necessary, referral to family planning services in order to prevent high-risk or unwanted pregnancies.

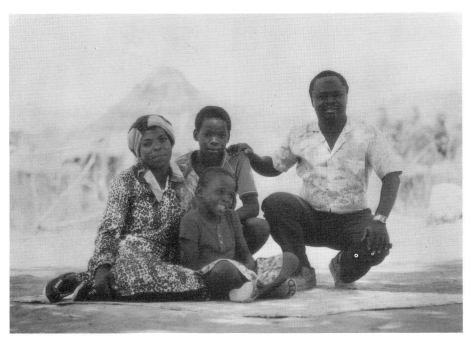

Reproductive health services should be targeted to families and communities, not only to women. (T. Kelly/WHO/19191)

Who. Parents of children brought for care; any woman or man of reproductive age receiving routine health services for any reason. Men and women should have joint responsibility for family planning, and health care providers need to advise men as well as women on family planning issues.

How and when. Assess by enquiry during routine visits for prenatal care and postpartum or well-baby care, as well as other routine health services. A confidential environment is essential. The home-based mother's record can be a useful tool in that it shows reproductive history, including gravidity, parity, birth outcome, and interpregnancy interval, indicating those persons who are in a high-risk category.

Resource levels required. Low for detection. Low (family planning education, provision of condoms or other barrier contraceptives), medium (provision of oral contraceptives and diaphragms, vasectomy) or high (tubal ligation) for intervention.

Recommendation on screening/early detection. Recommended as an adjunct to primary prevention; screening for risk of future unintended or high-risk pregnancies should be integrated into routine prenatal and postpartum care. "Opportunistic" screening and early detection are recommended as a part of all other health services including services for adults and services for children that present opportunities for communication with parents. While screening should be opportunistically integrated into routine health services, this approach will fail to reach those who do not use the health services. Population-based (in pre- and postnatal services) and opportunistic screening for the risk of unintended or high-risk pregnancy is recommended, but should be considered a minor adjunct to broad public education and the provision of safe, culturally acceptable, and financially accessible family planning services.

● Sexually transmitted diseases (STDs), including HIV infection

Why. Early detection of STDs, other than HIV infection, can prevent serious morbidity in infected persons and their partners and prevent further spread.

Who, how, and when. All pregnant women should be screened for STDs, including HIV infection if they are at high risk and give their informed consent (see page 67); postpartum screening is needed only if exposure since prenatal screening is suspected. Screening for STDs should be performed at frequent intervals for persons with a number of sexual partners or those exposed to a partner with a number of partners. Persons at high risk should be encouraged to seek screening as soon as possible after likely exposure. The frequency of screening for STDs among the general population depends on local epidemiological circumstances. In some places it is standard practice to screen any adult or sexually active young person for syphilis (by VDRL test on blood) on any hospital admission; the yield from this practice needs to be examined in the local context. Screening should always be accompanied by primary prevention efforts.

Resource levels required. Medium for screening, including pre-test counselling for HIV testing; medium to high for definitive diagnosis; medium for treatment with antibiotics at an early stage. Medium or high for treatment of HIV-positive individuals, including post-test counselling; low for counselling to prevent further spread of STDs, although there is no evidence that counselling of HIV-positive individuals leads to reduced transmission.

Recommendation on screening/early detection. Opportunistic screening, case-finding, and early detection are recommended as adjuncts to primary prevention through community-wide education on safe sexual practices and provision of condoms and spermicides (most spermicides increase the effectiveness of condoms in preventing STDs). Routine health services should include confidential enquiries regarding risks of sexually transmitted disease including HIV infection, and screening tests as indicated by the medical history (see page 112). For all STDs, including HIV infection, screening should be seen only as an adjunct to broad public education, beginning in adolescence, regarding primary prevention and indications for self-referral to a health centre for appropriate care, along with provision of low-cost barrier methods that decrease the risk of disease transmission and other efforts at primary prevention. See pages 67–69 and 113.

● **Cervical cancer**

Those at highest risk for cervical cancer, namely women aged 35–55, are generally not reached through family planning services or prenatal and postpartum care. Special outreach action is needed. Coverage of these women should take priority over excessive screening of younger women as part of family planning programmes (see page 131).

● **Reproductive hazards in the workplace or home**

Recommendation on screening. Recommendation uncertain. To prevent reproductive hazards in the workplace or home, particular emphasis must be placed on legislation, regulations, and their enforcement, as well as on public education. Screening does not appear to have an important role in the prevention of this category of health problem, although it may be desirable for health care providers to enquire, as the opportunity arises, about potential hazards in areas where exposure is common and a campaign of primary prevention is under way.

Care of the newborn[1]

As in the case of prenatal care, we have included under this heading some conditions whose identification may more precisely fit the broad category of early detection, rather than the narrower category of screening, because they represent pathological conditions with observable signs, such as low birth weight. Many such conditions that are important precursors of serious morbidity or mortality may go unrecognized by primary care workers or parents. This is especially so in places where access to services and the training of birth attendants are limited. The risk of such conditions being seen as within the normal spectrum is especially great where they are particularly common.

● **Low birth weight/prematurity**

Why. Low birth weight is the single best predictor of neonatal survival and is a significant risk factor in the postneonatal period. Low birth weight is not necessarily associated with clear signs of pathology in newborns and thus may not be obvious, especially in areas where its incidence is high and where home births are common. Detecting low birth weight can thus be

---

[1] The following publication was used extensively as a general reference for this section: Macfarlane et al. (1989).

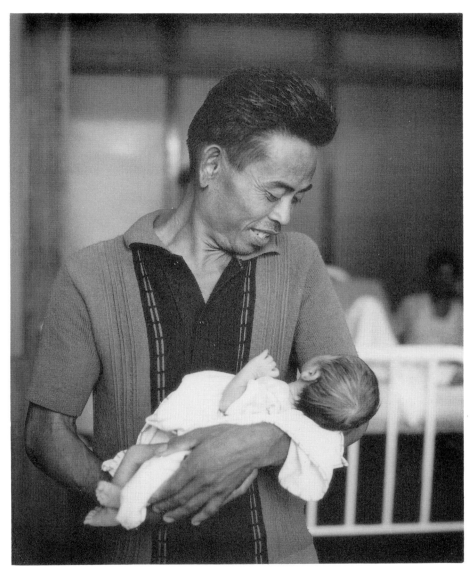

A proud father holds his newborn child. (P. Almasy/WHO/16571)

thought of as either early detection or screening. The detection of low birth weight should be undertaken as soon as possible after birth; many but not all low-birth-weight infants can be anticipated on the basis of prenatal factors. The aim is to identify newborn infants likely to need more intensive monitoring and treatment or support, often with referral to a health centre or hospital. In the early neonatal period, the care of a low-birth-weight baby at a centre equipped to care for high-risk infants is associated with a better outcome. Later, socioeconomic and psychosocial factors become the primary determinants of the outcome, rather than medical care *per se*. Primary care workers can provide additional psychosocial support and education on infant care in the neonatal and postneonatal periods, with referral as needed. Low birth weight is a good marker of risk even after infancy and throughout the early childhood period.

Who. All newborn infants.

How. Weighing is best, provided that the available scales are sufficiently sturdy to maintain their accuracy in difficult environmental conditions. Where home births are common, the scales have to be light enough to be

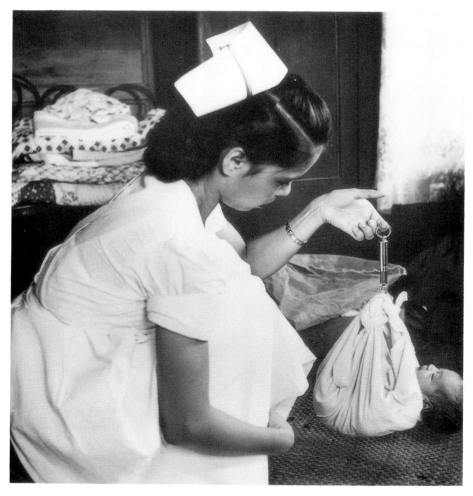

Weighing a newborn baby with hand-held portable scales.   (WHO/1362)

transported by a primary care worker. Where the literacy of primary care workers is limited, scales with culturally appropriate colour-coding have been used to indicate birth-weight ranges, so that actual numbers do not have to be read (WHO, 1984a). In some places it may be best to use scales that indicate simply whether a baby is under or over 2500 grams without giving a numerical reading (WHO, 1986b). If scales are not available, primary care workers can be trained to assess birth weight by measuring mid-arm or, preferably, chest circumference with specially marked tape-measures (WHO, 1987).

The birth weight (or whether a child is of normal or low birth weight) should be entered in a record that will guide the care of the child during infancy and the preschool years. The home-based child's record (HBCR), which was developed on the model of the home-based maternal record (HBMR), appears to be especially appropriate for use in a primary health care context. The linkage of the child's record with the mother's permits information to be carried over on maternal risk factors relevant in providing care for the child. Some home-based records developed for use by nonliterate mothers and health care workers contain pictures distinguishing normal from low-birth-weight babies.

Like the HBMR, the HBCR constitutes a simple guide to early detection of the most important risks. Furthermore, it provides the documentation needed for referral between the different levels within a health system, in a form that serves as an educational tool for parents as well as health workers.

When. As soon as possible after birth; risk assessment and preventive measures should be started in the prenatal period.

Resource levels required. Low for detection; low, medium, or high for intervention (additional support and more frequent monitoring by community health worker, or referral to more highly trained personnel for specialized care).

Recommendation on screening/early detection. Early detection is recommended as an adjunct to efforts to prevent low birth weight through prenatal and general health promotion. This includes providing family planning services and high quality, comprehensive prenatal care that addresses socioeconomic and psychosocial, as well as medical, risks. General health promotion includes multisectoral efforts focused on education, food supply, employment, and prevention of the use of tobacco, which appears to be a powerful determinant of low birth weight.

● **Maternal/household psychosocial and socioeconomic risks** that identify the "at-risk" child, or the child in an "at-risk" household (see partial list of factors, page 57).

Why. To provide additional support and monitoring to improve the outcome for the child, the mother, and other household members.

How. By enquiry, inspection of records, or assessment during routine home visit by health worker. Linkage of the mother's and child's home-based health records makes it possible to carry over important information on relevant risks. This information can be used to guide follow-up in the neonatal, postneonatal, and early childhood periods.

When. Ideally, at a home visit within a few days after birth.

Resource levels required. Low for screening; low or medium skill required for definitive diagnosis; low, medium, or high resources for intervention, depending on nature of problem.

Recommendation on screening/early detection. Screening and early detection recommended. Screening and early detection of household psychosocial and socioeconomic risks for the newborn should begin in the prenatal period.

Research priority. Validation of the effectiveness of methods using primary care workers.

● Congenital syphilis

Why. Congenital syphilis is quite common in certain populations (e.g., 7.5% of 200 babies screened in an intensive care unit in Lusaka (Bhat et al., 1982)) and its timely treatment prevents severe neurological sequelae.

How and when. Testing of cord blood collected at delivery.

Resource levels required. Medium technology levels for detection (cord blood VDRL and RPR) and treatment (parenteral antibiotics). Information system/communication resources needed for follow-up of positive results.

Recommendation on use of screening. Uncertain for testing new-born infants. Universal prenatal screening is recommended (see page 67). Neonatal as well as prenatal testing is desirable in very high-risk populations where maternal infection may have occurred after prenatal testing was performed. However, neonatal testing may be logistically difficult and is less important if there is universal coverage with prenatal testing and follow-up (Stray-Pedersen, 1983).

● Undescended testis

Why. Surgical treatment at the age of one year can reduce the risk of infertility; it may also lower the risk of testicular cancer (Macfarlane et al., 1989).

How. Physical examination.

When. Needs to be done by the age of one year; if both testes have descended at birth, no further screening is needed. Screening at birth may be desirable to identify those requiring further screening in infancy (see page 93).

Resource levels required. Medium for detection (no instruments required but staff need careful training and experience). High for intervention.

Recommendation on use of screening. Uncertain for neonatal screening, if resources are very limited and a reliable examination with appropriate follow-up cannot be assured for all. Essential to have reliable screening no later than age of one year.

● Congenital hypothyroidism

Why. Congenital hypothyroidism leads to serious sequelae, including severe mental retardation, which can be prevented if medical treatment is given within the first 1–2 months of life (USPSTF, 1989; Modell et al., 1991).

Who. Newborn infants in areas where iodine deficiency is common.

How and when. By thyroid function tests on cord blood collected at delivery; newborn cord-blood assay is less expensive than blood assay in pregnant women, and 24-hour urine assay in pregnant women is impractical. A review of experience in India in 1981 calculated costs as 29 US cents per test, and as $4.80 per case found, and acknowledged that these costs should be compared with those of universal iodine supplementation in areas of known deficiency, which were likely to be lower (Thompson et al., 1981). Further experience in India stressed the formidable organizational problems involved in ensuring adequate follow-up of results of cord-blood tests (Desai et al., 1987). A relatively inexpensive method has been developed in which birth attendants send samples of cord blood on special filter-paper to a central laboratory by mail in pre-addressed envelopes; this permits testing in populations where home births are the norm (Pandav & Kochupillai, 1985). While this method is less expensive than traditional ones, it requires a good communications infrastructure to ensure follow-up. Blood testing may be unacceptable in some cultures.

Resource levels required. Medium technology and moderate cost (primarily for tracking results/communications) for testing cord blood on filter-paper sent to central laboratory; medium or high for definitive diagnosis; low for intervention through iodine supplementation.

Recommendation on use of screening. Uncertain; depends on local conditions. Screening is not recommended in places with poor communications between the central laboratory and the primary care level. Alternative strategies emphasizing primary prevention through salt iodization in endemic areas and the early detection of goitre through physical examination of all pregnant women (by palpation) may be more rational in a primary health care context (see page 63).

- ## Congenital dislocation of the hip

Why. Untreated congenital dislocation of the hip leads to disability. Early detection and treatment are associated with improved outcome; non-surgical treatment may be possible.

How and when. The clinical examination of neonates for congenital dislocation of the hip, done as part of a routine newborn examination, may require highly trained personnel to perform the Ortolani-Barlow manoeuvre and test hip abduction and adduction (Macfarlane et al., 1989). This may not be possible in places with limited professional resources. The detection of hip dislocation in an older infant or toddler is easier and permanent impairment should still be preventable (see page 92).

Resource levels required. Medium for screening (low technology, but a highly skilled examiner); medium or high for definitive diagnosis; high for intervention (requires orthopaedic consultation, possibly surgery).

Recommendation on use of screening. Uncertain if resources are very limited. Recommended early in toddler period (around the age of two years). Detection is easier in a toddler, and disability is generally avoidable if the condition is detected early in the toddler stage.

- ## Treatable abnormalities of head circumference in the newborn

Why. To detect hydrocephalus or a subdural haematoma before brain damage occurs. Intervention requires neurosurgery (to insert shunt or evacuate haematoma).

How. There is great inter-examiner variability in measurement of head circumference by unskilled examiners; a special measuring-tape and training are required, as well as radiological facilities (computerized tomography) for definitive diagnosis, and neurosurgical treatment at hospital.

When. As part of a routine newborn examination, within 1–2 days after birth.

Resource levels required. Low to medium for initial screening; high or very high for definitive diagnosis; high or very high for intervention.

Recommendation on use of screening. Uncertain. Not as high a priority as recommended screening practices, because of difficulties in detection, the expense of intervention, and the rarity of the conditions sought. Not recommended unless facilities and personnel for definitive diagnosis and treatment are available for the entire population, and population-wide services for more common conditions have already been established.

- ## Asymptomatic cardiac abnormality

Why. To identify newborn infants with structural cardiac abnormalities before they become symptomatic, and to refer them for evaluation for surgical or medical therapy.

How. Auscultation with a stethoscope.

When. As part of a routine newborn examination, within 1–2 days after birth.

Resource levels required. Medium for screening, which will require a trained professional; even then, there may be many false positives resulting in the labelling of well children as sick; definitive diagnosis requires high or very high resources, including X-ray, echocardiography, and coronary arteriography which may not be available at the district hospital level. Treatment also involves considerable expense (surgical correction or long-term antibiotic therapy), which may be beyond district resources.

Recommendation on use of screening. Uncertain as regards screening where resources are very limited. Many abnormalities will produce some symptoms. All newborns should be examined for normal activity, behaviour, and appearance, with early detection and referral of symptomatic infants to more specialized personnel or centres. It is unclear what impact the early detection of asymptomatic conditions has in settings with severely limited resources for definitive diagnosis and treatment.

● Sickle-cell disease and other haemoglobinopathies

Why. For haemoglobinopathies other than sickle-cell disease, the purpose of neonatal testing is to permit genetic counselling on future reproductive decisions. The impact of information given soon after birth that can be used only for genetic counselling in the reproductive years is doubtful, without an intensive long-term follow-up that will be beyond the capacity of most services in developing countries. However, there is evidence that early detection of sickle-cell disease leads to more effective intervention with appropriate treatment of crises (USPSTF, 1989).

How, when, and resource levels required. Haemoglobin electrophoresis is performed on blood collected during newborn screening and possibly re-screening after a few months. The technique is moderately expensive, as is genetic counselling, which requires specialized training. Special tests to detect sickle-cell disease are less expensive, but skilled counselling is also required and treatment for repeated crises is hospital-based and expensive in the long term. Resource levels are high for detection and intervention for most haemoglobinopathies; medium for detection and medium or high for intervention for sickle-cell disease.

Recommendation on use of screening. Uncertain as regards screening for sickle-cell disease in high-prevalence populations; not recommended where there is an inadequate infrastructure for the treatment of all individuals affected (Griffiths, 1982). Screening for other haemoglobinopathies is not recommended as a priority.

Research priority. To develop effective community-based approaches to counselling and treatment for sickle-cell disease.

● **Phenylketonuria**

Why. Phenylketonuria incidence is estimated at 1 in 10 000 live births in the United Kingdom (Macfarlane et al., 1989); the results of large-scale screening in an area of China showed an incidence of 1 in 16 500 (Liu & Zuo, 1986). Untreated phenylketonuria is associated with severe mental retardation. Treatment consists of a strict diet and elimination of food sources containing phenylalanine. The effectiveness of counselling is not well documented, however, particularly in places where dietary choice is limited (USPSTF, 1989).

How and when. The test is ideally done by heel-prick at age 6–10 days; this may be logistically difficult with rural or marginal urban populations, especially since repeat tests are often needed (CTF, 1979).

Resource levels required. High (central laboratory) for detection; medium for intervention (uncertain effectiveness).

Recommendation on use of screening. Uncertain. Testing for this rare but devastating condition is controversial even in industrialized countries, because the cost is high relative to the yield. Testing for phenylketonuria in developing countries is especially problematic because it is expensive, and dietary choice is generally restricted.

● **Other inborn errors of metabolism**

Why. The outcome of some inborn errors of metabolism may be improved with treatment. These conditions are rare, however, and it has not been demonstrated that intervention before symptoms develop is superior to early detection of signs and symptoms.

How and when. Biochemical assays of blood or urine during neonatal period.

Resource levels required. High or very high for detection; variable for treatment, but generally high or very high, including highly specialized counselling.

Recommendation on use of screening. Not recommended. These conditions are extremely rare, detection is expensive, and the benefit of treatment in asymptomatic newborn infants is questionable. Screening for inborn errors of metabolism other than phenylketonuria is not recommended as standard practice in the USA, because of the low yield for a high cost (USPSTF, 1989).

● **Eye abnormalities**

Why. Eye development continues for several years after birth. Screening is done to identify newborn infants with eye disorders (other than those clearly observable on external physical observation without instruments) requiring medical or surgical treatment to ensure that eye development will not be impaired, and to determine if special precautions are needed to minimize learning disabilities.

How and when. Ophthalmoscopic examination for absence of red reflex, as part of routine examination of newborn (within 1–2 days after birth).

Resource levels required. Medium for screening; high for definitive diagnosis; high or very high for treatment.

Recommendation on use of screening. Uncertain in places where resources are highly constrained, because of the resource levels required for detection and treatment and the relative rarity of conditions for which early detection in the newborn would allow effective intervention. Not among the highest priorities for neonatal screening. Early detection of visual problems in preschool-age and school-age children is recommended; this requires education of parents and teachers and accessible, acceptable services.

CHAPTER 6

Screening in child health care

This chapter covers screening in care for infants (after the immediate neonatal period), children under 6 years of age, school-age children and adolescents; additional discussion of screening for communicable diseases among children as well as adults is covered in Chapter 7.

Care of infants and children under 6 years of age[1]

The home-based child's record (HBCR) appears to be an excellent tool to guide screening activities by health workers and to educate parents. It documents health risks and needs in a way that can facilitate referrals between

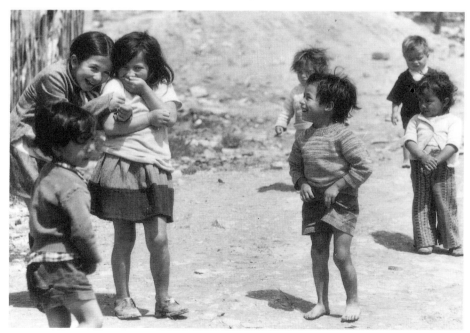

Primary care workers are often appropriately placed to screen young children.
(J. Littlewood/WHO/18354)

---

[1] In addition to the references listed in the footnote to page 49, Macfarlane et al. (1989) was an important general reference for this section.

different levels of care when necessary (Shah & Shah, 1981; Shah et al., 1988). The HBCR is a familiar concept, combining immunization records and growth curves with indicators of development at appropriate stages. Recent documents from the United Kingdom stress the importance of active enquiry regarding any parental concern about a child's health or development as a means of early detection that can replace many screening tests (Butler, 1989; Macfarlane et al., 1989).

The use of primary care workers to screen young children within well-child programmes is well established. Documents from the Working Party in the United Kingdom suggest that, given adequate training and supervision, paramedical "health visitors" could play an important part in screening preschool children for physical and developmental abnormalities (Butler, 1989; Hall, 1989b). A study in Nigeria in the mid-1970s demonstrated the capacity of public health nurses and community nurses (auxiliaries with training in midwifery and practical nursing) to screen preschool and school-age children for a variety of developmental and physical handicaps, but stressed the importance of adequate training and of realistic workloads in order to ensure quality (Okunade, 1980). A project in Denver, USA, in which health aides screened preschool children in extremely low-income families showed that those workers could accurately perform a variety of screening tests, including assessments of speech, hearing, vision, overall development, and dental caries (Dawson, 1976).

The screening of children for infectious diseases is discussed to a limited extent in this chapter. It is primarily covered in Chapter 7.

● **The "at-risk" infant or preschool child;** the infant/preschool child in the "at-risk" household (see discussion of household psychosocial and socio-economic risk factors in Chapter 5, page 57).

Why. In order to keep the "at-risk" child under close surveillance and increase promotional efforts aimed at the family; to refer the "at-risk" child for more specialized services if necessary. All low-birth-weight infants should be considered as being at elevated risk throughout the early childhood years (unless their early development indicates the absence of special risks), and their households should be the subject of special surveillance and promotional efforts.

How. By enquiry and a review of neonatal and prenatal history, checking especially for low birth weight or prematurity, or by routine home assessment by a health worker. By linking the HBCR and the HBMR, key maternal and neonatal risk factors that should guide the preventive and promotional care of the young child can be identified. Other medical, environmental, or psychosocial factors can be detected from the prenatal history and from home assessment. Care providers should ask parents whether they have particular worries about the child's health; this is an example of early detection. Inadequate immunization status for age may be a good indicator of a child generally at risk who could benefit from special support at the household level. Routine postpartum home visiting may provide a valuable opportunity for a trained health worker to make an assessment of household risk; subsequent visits can be targeted to households and infants at high risk.

When. At first well-baby check.

Resource levels required. Low for initial detection; complete assessment may require a medium or high level of training. Resources for intervention may be low, medium, or high, ranging from increased psychosocial support from primary care workers or increased socioeconomic support from community sources to referral for specialized services.

Recommendation on use of screening. Screening and early detection recommended. However, priority should be given to primary prevention through overall community-wide improvements in socioeconomic status, in the status of women, and in education.

Research priority. Developing and evaluating the effectiveness of methods of training and supervising primary care workers for the assessment and handling of psychosocial and socioeconomic risks.

● Immunization status

Why. To immunize against poliomyelitis, diphtheria, pertussis, tetanus, measles, mumps, and rubella, and against tuberculosis (BCG), hepatitis B, and possibly haemophilus influenza B, as indicated by local policies. Inadequate immunization status at different stages may also be an indicator of a child who is generally at risk.

How. By a review of the child's health record, which should contain the recommended schedule of immunizations. This can be done quickly by inspecting the home-based child's record or by using a checklist placed at the front of a clinical chart.

When. At every routine visit. The immunization schedule determines the timing of routine visits for well-child care and other screening. Immunization schedules vary from country to country, but BCG and hepatitis B vaccine are usually given at birth and other immunizations are initiated at the age of 1–2 months. Periodic community-wide immunization campaigns, in which primary care workers and volunteers perform a door-to-door "census" of immunization coverage and provide immunization to those who are not up-to-date, have been successful in reaching populations that do not regularly use health services.

Resource levels required. Low for detection (enquiry, review of record); low or medium for intervention (vaccination).

Recommendation on use of screening. Recommended. In communities with poor access to services, there should be an outreach programme to screen all young children for immunization status and correct any deficits, on a community-wide basis, not only among those using institutional health services. Schedules for immunization should determine the timing of most well-baby checks. At every visit for acute or preventive care, the opportunity should be taken to check immunization status in relation to recommended schedules.

• Monitoring of physical growth

Why. To intensify efforts to promote better nutrition among children with deficiencies, through education and food supplements if available. If screening demonstrates that nutritional problems are widespread in a community, it would be advisable to consider measures outside, as well as within, the health sector that could improve nutritional status.

How. Assessment by parents, health workers and other caregivers of whether or not a child is thriving. Documentation of child's growth curve (looking at the child's progress in relation to prior measurements, rather than in relation to others) may be a useful adjunct. The home-based child's growth card is a useful tool for guiding screening.

A variety of methods have been used for monitoring children's physical growth as a reflection of nutritional status as well as other factors (United Nations, 1986). Weight for age, height for age, and weight for height are most common as initial screening criteria, with arm circumference as an aid in classifying degrees of malnutrition. Various types of scales and calibrated devices for measuring height and body circumferences have been tested for use in developing countries (Trowbridge & Staehling, 1980; WHO, 1986b,c). The value of arm circumference measurement has been confirmed and is considered by some researchers to be not only reliable but easiest for primary care workers with limited training to perform (Smith, 1989). Screening by arm circumference has been found to detect a greater number of severely malnourished children at a younger age than screening by weight for height (Smith, 1989).

When. At each visit as determined by the immunization schedule.

Resource levels required. Low for screening; medium, high, or very high for definitive diagnosis if following up on metabolic disorders. Low, medium, high, or very high for treatment, depending on condition identified.

Recommendation on use of screening. Uncertain; early detection of inadequate weight gain recommended. There is concern not only about the inappropriateness of applying the same growth standards to diverse populations, but also about the lack of evidence that growth monitoring *per se* results in improved child health in many of the places where poor growth is particularly common (Tanner et al., 1987; Nabarro & Chinnock, 1988). The use of growth curves can lead to the classification of a certain percentage of the population as abnormal. Labelling children as growing poorly – even according to their own baseline – can produce anxiety and often feelings of guilt in parents, who may not be able to act to improve growth. Growth monitoring can be useful, if it is part of an overall assessment of whether or not a child is thriving and combined with an assessment of the psychosocial and socioeconomic risks in the particular household. However, the cost of population-wide screening and medical treatment should be balanced against that of a primary prevention programme aimed at improving nutritional status for the entire population, supplemented by early detection of poor growth, especially in children considered to be in "at-risk" households.

Primary prevention of nutritional deficiencies on a community-wide basis is preferable to investing resources in screening. Where supplements are available or counselling has been shown to be effective, it may be advisable to screen children for deficiencies in particular nutrients, such as vitamin A (Pratinidhi et al., 1987).

● Mental, neurological and psychosocial development

Why. To provide additional support and counselling to families of children with problems of development, and referral to any special services available in the community, health centre or district, in order to minimize impairments and their consequences. Counselling and referral may involve highly specialized diagnostic and treatment resources. However, emphasis should be placed on primary care measures at the community level, promotion of parents' skills in child-rearing according to local norms, and early stimulation of children's learning capacity. Teenage parents and parents isolated from their extended family may be in particular need of support.

How. Restandardization of the Denver Developmental Screening Test (DDST) for use in northern China has been the subject of an apparently successful large-scale study (Collaborative Study Group of Child Developmental Test, 1986). Such formal developmental testing is, however, expensive, and is not recommended as an initial screening technique by either the US Preventive Services Task Force (USPSTF, 1989) or the UK Working Party (Macfarlane et al., 1989). It seems rational for parents and primary care workers to assess a child's overall development routinely according to culturally appropriate milestones, e.g., speech, crawling, walking, dressing self, feeding self. The home-based child's health card can be a useful tool in developmental screening, with pictorial aids for assessing the milestones. Children found to have abnormalities on initial screening by primary care workers, or whose parents express concern about their development, should be referred for formal testing if the relevant diagnostic and treatment services are available on a population-wide basis.

When. Frequency will depend on culture-specific milestones for acquisition of skills. The immunization schedule would be a rational determinant of the developmental screening schedule, with a culturally appropriate milestone being selected for each stage.

Resource levels required. Low for detection by primary care workers guided by the pictorial symbols on the home-based child's record. Medium, high, or very high for definitive diagnosis and intervention by trained personnel.

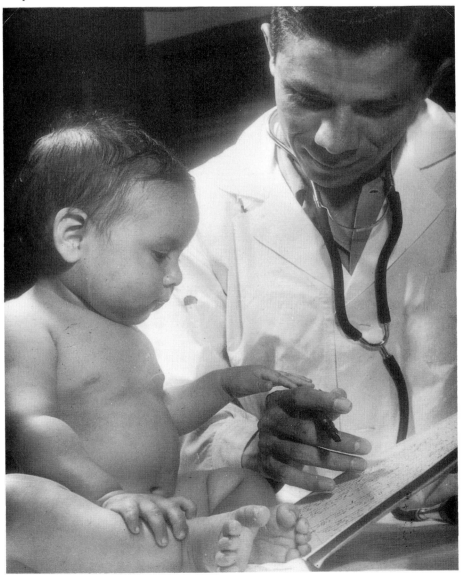

A doctor at a clinic in El Salvador informally assesses an infant's development during a well-baby visit. (WHO/3653)

Recommendation on use of screening/early detection. Screening and early detection are recommended, using simple culturally appropriate milestones that can be assessed by primary care workers. Formal developmental testing is not recommended. Parents and child care workers should be taught to refer for evaluation any child who is not progressing according to community standards, and health care providers should be trained to ask parents and other care-givers about any subject of concern during routine well-baby and well-child visits. Even where resources are not available for definitive diagnosis and specialized intervention, primary care workers can train family members and care providers to give special attention and support in order to minimize impairments and prevent child abuse.

Research priority. Developing primary care methods of screening and intervention.

● Congenital dislocation of hip

Why. Early detection and treatment are associated with improved outcome. Treatment will generally involve referral to at least the health centre level and, if surgical treatment is necessary, to the district hospital.

How and when. Assessment before a child is walking may require a highly trained nurse or a doctor to perform the Ortolani-Barlow manoeuvre and test hip abduction and adduction. This may not be possible where professional resources are limited. In addition, the test is not useful after the age of 3 months (Hall, 1989). It may be possible, however, to train primary care workers to assess a toddler's gait at the routine visits for immunization; leg asymmetry, failure to walk by 18 months, or abnormal gait may be used as initial screening factors for congenital dislocation of the hip in the toddler (Macfarlane et al., 1989).

Resource levels required. Low for detection; medium or high for definitive diagnosis; high for intervention.

Recommendation on use of screening. Recommended in toddlers; difficult to test in younger children.

● Visual problems (strabismus, amblyopia, defects in visual acuity)

Why. Correction of strabismus (squint) or amblyopia before the age of 3–4 years can prevent permanent blindness. Treatment will involve the services of a specialist at the district hospital level. As regards defects in visual acuity, there seems to be no clear evidence that screening of preschool children results in a better outcome than diagnosis at school entry (Hall, 1989).

When. Ideally, around the age of 3 years. Screening test may be done along with routine immunizations at 18 or 24 months of age in places where an additional routine check-up at 3 years is unlikely.

How. Inspection of eyes for obvious abnormalities; cover–uncover test; examination of extra-ocular movements. It should be possible to train primary care workers to perform these tests (Dawson et al., 1976). However, the UK Working Party commented on the need for considerable skill and proper training to detect squint (Hall, 1989). Reports from Nigeria have stressed the need to instruct primary care workers in formal methods of assessing vision in preschool children (Okunade, 1980). A report from Israel describes the use of a technique called "rapid retinoscopy" for screening preschool children for strabismus and amblyopia; this is less costly and requires less highly trained personnel than ophthalmoscopy (Friedman et al., 1983). However, established screening tests for amblyopia and strabismus do not require equipment, and neither the Canadian Task Force nor the UK Working Party recommended ophthalmoscopy or retinoscopy for screening for visual deficits in preschool children (CTF, 1979; Macfarlane et al., 1989; Hall, 1989).

Resource levels required. Low or medium for screening; medium or high for definitive diagnosis; medium, high, or very high for intervention.

Recommendation on use of screening. Recommended to screen for strabismus and amblyopia in preschool children. There is no primary prevention for these visual problems. Screen at immunization visits and promote early detection by educating the population to seek services if children have an abnormal appearance or functional difficulties. Screening for visual acuity is not recommended until school entry.

● Hearing problems

Why. To detect correctable defects before language is impaired, or provide special training if the defect is uncorrectable.

How. There is no accurate screening test. Formal audiometry is difficult and expensive in the case of preschool children.

Resource levels required. Medium or high for definitive diagnosis. For treatment: low (supportive measures to minimize impact of handicap); low to medium (treatment of otitis); high or very high (hearing aid or surgery).

Recommendation on use of screening. Routine screening is not recommended, but early detection of hearing problems should be encouraged by educating parents to seek services for any source of concern and by routinely asking them about any concerns as part of routine well-child care. Children with suspected defects should be referred for medical evaluation as early as possible to prevent educational difficulties.

● Undescended testis

Why. If left untreated, this condition may lead to infertility (especially if it is bilateral) and increased risk of testicular cancer. Although the benefits of early intervention are not firmly established (Macfarlane et al., 1989), surgery is the current standard intervention where the resources are available.

Who and when. All males at the age of one year, unless earlier screening has shown that both testes have descended. Screening for undescended testes should ideally be performed at birth on all male babies, but this requires a skilled examiner and many children found abnormal at birth will be normal by the age of one without intervention. If the neonatal examination finds the child to be normal, no further screening is required. If one or both testes are undescended at birth, screening should be repeated at the time of each immunization, and a child whose testes are undescended by the age of one should be referred for surgery.

Resource levels required. Low or medium for screening; medium for definitive diagnosis; high for treatment (surgery).

Recommendation on use of screening. Recommended at age of one year where resources exist for referral for surgery.

● **Treatable abnormalities of head circumference in infant**

Why. Increased intracranial pressure can have disastrous consequences and, in many instances, is treatable (hydrocephalus and subdural haematoma). Neurosurgical intervention (shunting or evacuation of haematoma) is needed.

How and resource levels required. Screening requires special measuring-tape and training; there are likely to be many false positives. Definitive diagnosis is expensive. Resources needed are low or medium for screening, and high or very high for definitive diagnosis and intervention.

When. Especially during and soon after neonatal period.

Recommendation on use of screening. Uncertain. Not as high a priority as recommended screening practices, because of difficulties in detection, the expense of intervention, and the rarity of the conditions sought. Not recommended as a priority unless facilities and personnel for definitive diagnosis and treatment are available for every infant discovered to have an abnormality.

● **Asymptomatic bacteriuria**

Why. Screening has been performed for asymptomatic bacteriuria in young children but a connection between the condition and subsequent health problems has not been established.

Recommendation on use of screening. Not recommended. The US Preventive Services Task Force recommends screening preschool children but notes that "there have been few studies proving that preschool urinalyses result in lower morbidity from recurrent infection or less renal damage" (USPSTF, 1989). The UK Working Party recommends against screening for this condition in this age group, noting the high expense of accurate testing and its low yield (Macfarlane et al., 1989).

● Subclinical iron deficiency anaemia and lead poisoning

Why. Infants and preschool children have often been screened for subclinical iron deficiency anaemia, but its significance is unclear. Moderately severe iron deficiency anaemia (haemoglobin $\leq$ 100 g/l) in infants is associated with long-term developmental disadvantage (Lozoff et al., 1991). However, microcytic anaemia may be a marker for lead poisoning; adverse health effects of lead on young children have been demonstrated at very low blood levels. Environmental lead poisoning is a particular problem for children exposed to automobile exhaust fumes (as in crowded urban areas) or to buildings with lead paint.

Recommendation on use of screening. Not recommended. Efforts would be better concentrated on community-wide promotion of better nutrition and sanitation (to prevent intestinal parasitoses) and the prevention of lead poisoning through environmental protection measures (legislation to prevent the use of leaded petrol and lead-based paints, and programmes to remove environmental lead).

● Asymptomatic rheumatic heart disease and other asymptomatic cardiac abnormalities

Why. To give long-term antibiotic prophylaxis to prevent further damage to heart valves from repeated streptococcal infection. To discover defects before they become symptomatic.

How. Accurate screening can be done only by a highly skilled professional health worker (Finau & Taylor, 1988). The many false positives recorded on clinical examination carry the danger of labelling well children as sick. In many places, the expense of definitive diagnosis (echocardiography) and long-term antibiotic prophylaxis for those in greatest need will be beyond the means of the health services.

Resource levels required. Medium for screening by auscultation with a stethoscope, but many false positives; high or very high for definitive diagnosis (examination by specialist, echocardiography, electrocardiography, angiography); medium (long-term antibiotic prophylaxis), high, or very high (cardiac surgery) for treatment.

Recommendation on use of screening. Not recommended as a priority. Efforts would be better spent on ensuring the accessibility of health services to prevent rheumatic heart disease and provide early diagnosis and treatment for those showing symptoms. The benefits of treatment of asymptomatic cardiac abnormalities other than long-term prophylaxis for rheumatic heart disease are unclear.

● **Elevated blood cholesterol**

Why. High blood cholesterol levels are associated with increased incidence of coronary artery disease in adulthood.

Recommendation on use of screening. Not recommended. The condition is very rare in the general child population. Testing is expensive and the likelihood of benefit very small. Screening may be indicated where there is a strong family history of hypercholesterolaemia or early cardiac disease. Efforts would be better spent on community-wide promotion of healthy diets, adequate exercise, and other measures to prevent coronary artery disease, e.g., the prevention of tobacco use and alcohol abuse.

● **High blood pressure**

Recommendation on use of screening. Not recommended in infants and preschool children. High blood pressure is very rare in young children (Macfarlane et al., 1989). A study in Israel found no hypertension among more than 1500 children aged 5–14 years (Zadik et al., 1987). Efforts would be better spent on community-wide primary prevention of risk of ischaemic heart disease and stroke (see also page 106).

Care of school-age children and adolescents

General comments

After school entrance, there are a limited number of medical conditions for which routine screening is an important part of health care. Early detection of psychosocial, developmental, and socioeconomic risks should receive the highest priority during the school years. At the most general level, the objective of screening all children should be thought of as identifying the "at-risk" child, which includes the child in an "at-risk" household. School-based providers of health care may find information on the household to be more limited for the school-age group than it is for younger children, who must be accompanied on their visits for care by a parent or other member of the household. Mass screening of children on entering school provides an opportunity to review preschool (maternal and infant) records, which should contain information on the risk status of households. After that, however, properly trained teachers should be in an excellent position to detect evidence of problems in schoolchildren's overall development and well-being. This comes under the broad heading of early detection (of a manifest problem) rather than screening proper (i.e., uncovering problems for which there are as yet no recognizable signs or symptoms).

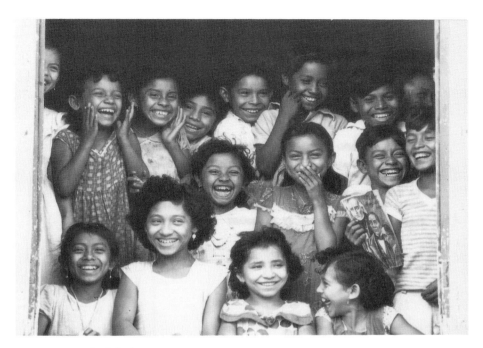

Schoolchildren in Mexico.   (P. Almasy/WHO/8515)

Teachers and care providers should be alert to signs that a child or adolescent is at high risk, e.g., frequent injuries, a history of child abuse or neglect in the household, or a precarious social situation at home (domestic violence, alcohol-related problems). They should also look for signs of depression in adolescents, including violent or self-destructive behaviour, and pay special attention to those who have frequent acute illness or chronic illness, or who have just been in hospital. Poor school performance, behavioural problems, and poor attendance are all indicators of a high-risk child. Children identified as at high risk will require more intensive surveillance than others, as well as special screening schedules, not covered here.

In the case of children or adolescents not at school or living where school-based screening is not feasible for other reasons, most screening should be provided by primary care workers trained in the relevant techniques. The routine screening of children not at school will be difficult, and the opportunities for intervention may be limited owing to the socioeconomic conditions responsible for their not attending school in the first place.

Potential uses of screening in the care of school-age children and adolescents

● **Problems of growth and development,** including physical, neurological, mental, and psychosocial development

Why. To detect children who are not thriving and developing normally and refer them for further evaluation and follow-up. Follow-up does not necessarily require the services of highly specialized personnel. It may include community-based interventions at the primary care level, e.g., special attention from teachers and families to minimize learning difficulties or deal with emotional problems affecting development.

Who. All school-age children and adolescents.

How and when. All sources agree on the importance of monitoring growth and development at the time of school entrance (around the age of 5–6 years). Preschool records should be reviewed at that time. The United Kingdom Child Health Surveillance Programme recommends checking and recording height on a centile chart on school entrance, with further checks during the school years only if a particular concern arises; physical examination should be carried out only if there is a specific reason for concern. The Canadian Task Force recommended checking height, weight, and head, arm, and chest circumferences on school entrance and once more around the ages of 10–11 years. However, this was primarily for screening for hormonal problems, which may be too rare, and whose definitive diagnosis and treatment may be too expensive, to warrant high priority for inclusion in routine screening in a primary health care context.

WHO has produced guidelines on the monitoring of physical growth and development in developing countries (WHO, 1986b,c). The home-based child's record is an excellent tool for the monitoring of growth and development throughout the school years by trained primary care personnel.

It is to be hoped that children with nutritional problems will have been identified during infancy and the preschool years and will already be under special surveillance. It would therefore seem rational for mass screening to check and record heights and weights (if scales are available) to be carried out at school entrance and for measurements to be repeated only if there are grounds for concern. Locally appropriate standards can be used but the greatest emphasis should be placed on detecting the child who is not growing at an adequate rate according to her or his own baseline, rather than those who do not conform to absolute norms of height or weight. Primary care workers or teachers should be able to carry out such screening with proper training. Because problems of physical growth related to nutritional status would be expected to be more prevalent in poorer countries, more frequent screening may be desirable in these countries; this should, however, be done only if there are resources not only for screening but for effective intervention. For example, where widespread growth problems are largely due to endemic parasitism, community-wide efforts at preventing exposure may be more worth while than efforts to identify all those affected, whose antiparasitic treatment would have only a transient effect at best (Tanner et al., 1987).

The Canadian Task Force recommended mass screening for behavioural and developmental problems on school entrance, with further screening in school-age children "if warranted by earlier assessments". The UK Working Party was not in favour of formal screening for psychiatric or behavioural problems. Both groups recommended enquiry about sources of concern to parents as the mechanism for screening psychosocial development on school entrance. Language use, motor skills, and social interaction of children starting school should be routinely assessed by health workers or teachers. Many children's preschool health records specify developmental milestones and can thus guide assessment. Once children enter school, their school performance should indicate their mental development and point to any behavioural or learning disorders. Teachers should be trained to assess psychosocial development as a part of routine periodic assessment of children. In addition, during each visit for routine care, parents should be asked about any aspect of their child's psychosocial, as well as physical, development that is causing them concern; this fits an early detection model.

Resource levels required. Low for initial detection by teachers or primary care workers; medium or high for definitive diagnosis. Low, medium, high, or very high for intervention, depending on the nature of the problem. Some problems may be addressed by providing additional psychosocial or economic support for the family or food supplements for the child.

Recommendation on screening/early detection. Screening of overall development recommended on school entrance, with further assessments if concern is expressed by teachers or parents. The routine formal growth monitoring or developmental testing of school-age children is not recommended as a priority. Resources are better spent on primary prevention by promoting the overall socioeconomic development of the community and improving education and the status of women, as well as training teachers to detect potential problems of development at an early stage and make appropriate referrals.

Research priority. To develop accurate inexpensive ways for primary care workers or teachers to assess problems of overall physical and psychosocial development and address such problems, making optimum use of the resources locally available.

● Immunization status

Why. To bring immunization status up to date in relation to age. Inadequate immunization status indicates lack of access to care or inappropriate use of the available services and may be an indicator of an at-risk child or household that needs to be targeted for more intensive preventive and promotional follow-up.

Who. All school-age children and adolescents.

How. Enrolment in school should involve review of home-based records; a record should be created for each child who does not have a vaccination record.

When. On school entrance, all immunizations should be brought up to date according to local or national schedules. Tetanus booster (preferably in tetanus/diphtheria form) is recommended around the age of 15 years (assuming the previous booster shot was given around the age of 5), or 10 years after completion of the initial series. If resources are particularly limited, priority for revaccination (and hence for screening) should be given to girls near, or at, reproductive age (to prevent neonatal tetanus) and to anyone engaged in high-risk work. The Canadian Task Force recommended screening of all girls around the age of 10–11 years for a history of rubella immunization (by enquiry, checking titre where uncertain) and vaccinating those not previously immunized (CTF, 1979). The use of home-based records should provide adequate information on immunization status, preventing the need for checking titres and reducing the number of unnecessary revaccinations. Measles reimmunization is recommended on school entrance and may be especially important in developing countries where children are generally vaccinated against measles before they are one year old, or where potential problems in maintaining the cold chain make revaccination advisable.

Resource levels required. Low for detection; low for intervention (vaccination).

Recommendation on use of screening. Recommended as a priority on school entrance and at appropriate stages according to local schedules. Detection and intervention are inexpensive. Immunization against common childhood illnesses is of proven benefit.

● Visual problems

Why. Refractive defects are common in children and adolescents. A 1983 study in China (Province of Taiwan) cited a myopia prevalence of 13–27% in primary schools, 28–69% in junior high schools, and 79–89% in high schools; the study was "nationwide", but the numbers in the sample were not specified (Taiwan Department of Health, 1988). The goal of screening is to provide corrective lenses and thus prevent learning difficulties. Even where corrective lenses are not available, screening could lead to simple precautions to minimize learning difficulties, such as seating those with decreased visual acuity closest to the blackboard. Special screening may be needed in areas where vitamin A deficiency is prevalent and supplements can be given (Pratinidhi et al., 1987).

Who. All school-age children and adolescents.

How. Teachers or health workers can be trained to assess visual acuity with the use of a simple chart (pictorial at school entrance; Snellen-type during school years). Teachers should also be trained to spot children with reading difficulties and refer them for formal screening by trained health workers. Pratinidhi et al. (1987) discussed the validation of tests to improve the detection of visual manifestations of vitamin A deficiency in India. Another group in New Delhi suggested that primary school teachers could play a major role in the detection of several eye conditions, including infections and nutritional deficiencies as well as refractive errors (D'Souza et al., 1987).

When. Screening on school entrance is generally recommended. The United Kingdom Child Surveillance Programme recommends routine visual acuity checks at the ages of 8, 11, and 14 years (Macfarlane et al., 1989). The US Preventive Services Task Force does not make any recommendation on the subject, and the Canadian Task Force considers such checks as optional (CTF, 1979). The study in China (Province of Taiwan) cited above indicated a markedly increased prevalence of myopia with increasing age (Taiwan Department of Health, 1988). In a large study in the USA, 18% of children with normal vision at the age of 7 were found to have visual defects when rescreened at the age of 16 (Barnes, 1975); this suggests the advisability of at least one further screening after the preschool screening.

Resource levels required. Low for detection; medium for definitive diagnosis of refractive errors; low or medium for intervention.

Recommendation on use of screening. Recommended.

● Hearing problems

Why. Routine screening of schoolchildren for hearing problems has been practised in many industrialized countries. However, there is no clear evidence of benefit from early intervention in asymptomatic children. Teachers and parents should be taught to refer children with difficulty in hearing for evaluation; this is an example of early detection rather than screening as strictly defined. Timely intervention ranges from the treatment of chronic otitis to providing a hearing aid, or seating the child in a classroom in such a way as to minimize learning difficulties (e.g., close to the teacher), as well as training parents and other family members in simple techniques to improve communication with a hearing-impaired child.

How. No accurate screening test has been validated. Routine mass audiometry produces many false positives, resulting in children being labelled abnormal and considerable expense to make a definitive diagnosis.

In developed countries, the lack of a sufficiently specific test suitable for mass screening, the expense of definitive diagnosis and treatment, and the lack of clear evidence for the benefits of treatment in asymptomatic persons have led to the conclusion that screening for hearing problems is not suitable for mass application. Formal screening for hearing problems should therefore not be carried out except in high-risk groups; clearly, testing is indicated where there are clinical reasons for suspecting a problem (CTF, 1979; USPSTF, 1989) but this is not an example of screening.

Particular conditions in some countries or areas may warrant a different approach. Hearing deficits may be especially common in areas of endemic iodine deficiency (Wang & Yang, 1985); primary prevention should be the highest priority in such areas. Extremely high rates of middle-ear disease have been found on screening of schoolchildren in the USA who are recent immigrants from south-east Asia; this is possibly related to previous poor access to medical care and difficult socioeconomic conditions (Corth & Harris, 1984). A thoughtful review article by McPherson & Holborow (1988) suggests that screening schoolchildren for hearing loss may be more important in developing countries, where children may have had less contact with health services and are thus more likely to have significant undetected problems.

McPherson & Holborow make a case for "the importance of a practical assessment of local conditions and of avoiding preconceived procedures based on other cultures". They discuss the importance of an adequate health infrastructure for treatment as a precondition for establishing screening. "For example, in some places, while basic treatment for school children with otitis media can be arranged, no hearing aids are available. In such a situation, a screening programme that involves considerable health worker time in detecting sensorineural deficits may not be appropriate. Where hearing aids are not available a more realistic scheme might involve a simple categorization of a child's hearing for the benefit of parents and teachers. This alone may significantly improve his educational prospects. A screening procedure that allows for such factors may be quite different to those followed in developed nations."

They describe a procedure developed to screen children in the Gambia, which used only a series of questions to the child and to his or her teacher; children failing any of the questions on the initial screen then underwent otoscopy by a trained observer. Audiometry was not used. "Local health workers could initiate treatment of children referred. Those who passed were given a further test that checked their ability to perform simple commands without visual cues at a normal conversational level. The test used no expensive equipment and was designed to be carried out in normal school background noise. It was not designed to find actual threshold levels, merely to detect children with hearing problems serious enough to make them disadvantaged at school. Hearing aids were not available for distribution so more detailed studies were not required for rehabilitation purposes. The teachers and parents of children who failed the hearing screen were notified. Teachers were made aware that such students needed favourable seating in classes and extra attention. The use of hearing tactics for good communication was explained."

Resource levels required. Low for early detection by teachers or parents; medium or high for formal screening and high or very high for definitive diagnosis and treatment by specialist; medium for treatment of chronic otitis with antibiotics, high for insertion of ventilating tube.

Recommendation on screening/early detection. Routine formal screening is not recommended as a priority at this time. The early detection of possible hearing problems, or of overall learning or developmental problems, is recommended; this will rely on the education of teachers and on eliciting and responding to parental expressions of concern. Hearing can then be formally assessed among children about whom concern exists. Teachers should be trained to recognize schoolchildren with apparent hearing defects or with abnormalities of speech development.

● Oral health problems

Recommendation on use of screening. Not recommended as a priority. The Canadian Task Force recommends an annual oral/dental examination by a trained health worker from the age of 12 years. The US Preventive Services Task Force recommends oral health counselling at each routine visit and does not recommend routine mass screening. In developing countries, children have fewer caries and more gingival and periodontal disease than in industrialized countries (MH LeClercq, personal communication, 1989). In a primary health care context, fluoridation and mass public education to promote oral hygiene appear to be higher priorities than the dental screening of school-age children.

● Sexually transmitted diseases (STDs), including HIV infection, in sexually active adolescents. Screening for STDs is discussed in Chapter 5 (page 75) and Chapter 7 (page 112), but issues of special relevance to adolescents are considered here.

Why. Sexually active adolescents who tend to have a number of different partners or partners with a number of different partners are at especially high risk of STDs. Unmarried teenagers may be unlikely to seek care, even when symptoms appear, because they fear parental disapproval. Early detection and treatment of most sexually transmitted infections can prevent serious morbidity, infertility, and further spread.

Who. Sexually active adolescents of both sexes who have heterosexual relations and males who have homosexual relations.

How. Ensure that screening and treatment are carried out in a confidential and non-judgemental educational environment (Braveman & Toomey, 1987); provide education and support for prevention and treatment. Do not assume that all adolescents are heterosexual. School-based health centres, where culturally acceptable, offer important opportunities for the preventive and promotional care of adolescents, including confidential care when it is a question of reproductive health. Care providers in general medical or paediatric services need to be trained in ensuring confidentiality when caring for adolescents. Legislative issues (secular or religious) may be important obstacles (Paxman & Zuckerman, 1987).

When. Although local resources may make this infeasible, annual screening of sexually active adolescents has been recommended, by routine serological testing for syphilis and by cervical culture for gonorrhoea in girls. Cervical screening of girls for chlamydia should be done in high-prevalence areas, if resources permit; otherwise include presumptive treatment for chlamydia when treating gonorrhoea, syphilis, or other STDs in areas where chlamydia is known to be prevalent. Some sources have suggested routine testing of urine of asymptomatic males for pyuria, as an initial screen for gonorrhoea and chlamydia. Direct tests for chlamydia in urine have recently become available. Advantage can be taken of visits for other reasons to screen for prevalent local pathogens, as indicated by the exposure history; providers of care to adolescents should, as a matter of routine, make enquiries about sexual activity and advise on the use of barrier methods.

Resource levels required. Screening for STDs requires resources for initial screening at the health centre level and may require laboratory facilities at the district hospital level (VDRL testing). Resources needed are generally medium for screening; medium or high for definitive diagnosis; low or medium for treatment of all infections except HIV (see discussion of HIV screening page 67 and page 113).

Recommendation on use of screening. Routine screening (including educating the population at risk to seek screening) and "opportunistic" screening of high-risk groups are recommended. Universal confidential voluntary screening for common STDs, including HIV infection, among sexually active adolescents (heterosexuals, bisexuals, and gay males). Screening with treatment is a minor adjunct to primary prevention through providing education on safe sexual practices and making barrier methods accessible. High-risk groups (including gay and bisexual men and their sexual and close household contacts) should be vaccinated against hepatitis B; repeated testing of high-risk groups for infection is not rational once they have been vaccinated (and, ideally, their immune status established by antibody examination).

● Risk of pregnancy in school-age children

Why. Any adolescent under 18 years of age who becomes pregnant is at high risk of a miscarriage or of reduced quality of life as a young parent (limited schooling and economic opportunities, curtailment of freedom). Children of young adolescent parents without adequate resources from an extended family are at increased risk of suboptimal overall development.

Who, how, and when. When seen for health care, all adolescents should be asked routinely, in an atmosphere of trust and with explicit guarantees of confidentiality, whether they are sexually active. All sexually active hetero-

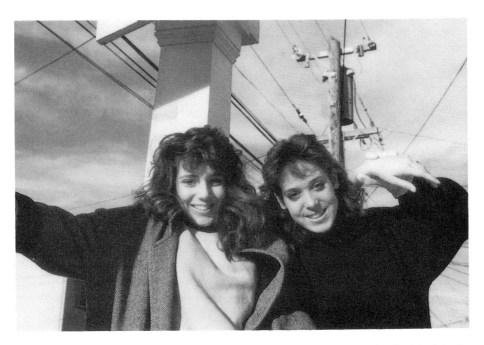

Increasing urbanization and industrialization are associated with changing health risks for adolescents.

sexual or bisexual adolescents should be asked whether they are using any form of contraception as well as protection against STDs. This should be done every time an adolescent has contact with the health services, whatever the reason, unless he or she is seen frequently for other reasons; if the person is seen frequently, the question should be asked at least every 6 months. Males as well as females should be asked, and family planning should be seen as the responsibility of both partners. This fits an "opportunistic" screening model. Confidential services for adolescents may be difficult to provide in a family-oriented culture; school-based services dealing with family planning may be unacceptable in many societies.

Resource levels required. Low for detection of risk; low or medium for intervention (education on safe sexual practices; prescription of an appropriate birth control method, taking into account risk of STDs as well as pregnancy).

Recommendation on use of screening. "Opportunistic" screening is recommended, but this should be seen as a minor adjunct to primary prevention through community-wide education beginning at an early age, together with providing universal access to safe, effective, and acceptable methods of family planning in a confidential atmosphere.

● Subclinical iron deficiency anaemia

Not recommended for general nonpregnant population. Routine screening of well school-age children for anaemia is not recommended by any of the authorities reviewed, because of lack of evidence of the clinical significance of mild anaemia without symptoms or signs. Pregnant teenagers should be screened for anaemia (see page 62).

● Scoliosis

Screening girls for scoliosis early in the period of rapid growth (puberty) has been widely practised. However, formal screening is not recommended, apart from inspection for obvious deformity, because of the lack of a sufficiently specific screening technique, the high cost of definitive diagnosis, and poor evidence of the effectiveness of treatment for scoliosis (CTF, 1979, 1984; Li et al., 1985; Huang et al., 1988; Macfarlane et al., 1989). Early detection is recommended (observation by teachers or parents of abnormal gait or uneven shoulder or hip height).

● High blood pressure

Why. High blood pressure may be common in adolescents in certain populations (e.g., in Africa). High blood pressure in childhood or youth places an individual at extremely high risk of ischaemic heart disease in adult life. Treatment is costly, however, and requires intensive long-term follow-up, education, and support.

Who. The US Preventive Services Task Force recommended screening of all children once between the ages of 13 and 18 (USPSTF, 1989), whereas the Canadian Task Force (CTF, 1979) did not recommend blood pressure screening for children or teenagers. A study in Israel of 1554 schoolchildren aged 5–14 years found no high blood pressure (Zadik et al., 1987). It appears rational to screen adolescents in populations known to have a high prevalence, but only if there are resources for appropriate follow-up. Otherwise, concentrating resources on policy changes and public education to promote healthy eating, exercise, and abstention from smoking should have higher priority as a preventive strategy than one that includes screening of children.

How. Measurement of blood pressure with a cuff and stethoscope. There should be no diagnosis or labelling unless abnormal values are registered on at least three consecutive readings.

Resource levels required. Low or medium for detection. Medium level of technology for intervention, but long-term treatment, including monitoring, medication, and visits, may be very expensive.

Recommendation on use of screening. Not recommended. Emphasis should be placed on the primary prevention of ischaemic heart disease through community-wide prevention of tobacco use and alcohol abuse and the promotion of exercise and a low-salt, low-fat diet.

● Elevated blood cholesterol

Recommendation on use of screening. Not recommended. Primary prevention of risk factors for ischaemic heart disease should be emphasized for the whole population (see discussion of cholesterol screening, page 96).

● Tuberculosis

Recommendation on use of screening/early detection. Screening is not recommended for asymptomatic persons in populations where BCG vaccination is routine and tuberculin testing is therefore not helpful. Where BCG vaccination is not routinely performed, tuberculin screening of children and adolescents in areas where tuberculosis may be a problem is recommended every two years. Routine X-ray screening is not recommended for asymptomatic persons, even in areas of relatively high prevalence (Aluoch et al., 1984; Gottridge et al., 1989; Kan, 1981; Krivinka et al., 1974; Stewart, 1966). Higher priorities for prevention include improvements in socioeconomic status, nutrition, and living conditions, together with early detection through mass public education on the importance of seeking care for persistent cough or haemoptysis, and training of health workers to look for signs and symptoms (case-finding) (see page 114).

● Asymptomatic bacteriuria

Recommendation on use of screening. Not recommended. The US Preventive Services Task Force did not recommend screening of school-age children (unless pregnant); there is no evidence of the value of screening for this condition among nonpregnant populations. Studies of the prevalence of asymptomatic bacteriuria in developing countries have shown rates similar to those recorded in developed countries (Badami & Deodhar, 1976; Elegbe et al., 1987). Screening for asymptomatic bacteriuria is recommended for pregnant women, including adolescents (see page 65).

● Schistosomiasis of urinary tract

Why. Schistosomiasis infection in childhood is a major cause of bladder cancer in adults. Although the infection is curable, reinfection will occur in the absence of major environmental measures.

Who. All school-age children and adolescents in endemic areas where efforts at primary prevention are under way.

How. Gross inspection of afternoon specimens of terminal urine stream has been used as an initial screen where resources are too limited to permit the use of reagent strips for initial screening (Cooppan et al., 1987; Mott et al., 1985; Sarda et al., 1986). Recent reports from a rural district in the United Republic of Tanzania describe a promising two-step approach, in which first-stage screening is based on a simple questionnaire regarding gross haematuria. The questionnaire is given out by teachers to primary school-children. Schools found to have low prevalence according to the question-naire are excluded from further screening; validation studies of the ques-tionnaire indicated a high negative predictive value (generally over 90%), i.e., few false negatives. Second-stage screening involves use of reagent strips to test for haematuria at the schools ascertained on the questionnaire to be at high risk (Lengeler et al., 1991a,b; Cooppan et al., 1987).

Resource levels required. Low for screening; medium for definitive diag-nosis; low or medium for intervention in an individual, but treatment is ineffective if re-exposure occurs.

Recommendation on use of screening. Uncertain in high-prevalence areas. First priority should be primary prevention. Effectiveness of early detection is uncertain where re-exposure is likely to occur.

- **Cancer screening of adolescents**

Testicular cancer. Testicular cancer is treatable if detected early. Self-examination of testicles may be helpful in improving early detection, but this has not been confirmed. Screening is not recommended as a priority for the general population, because of lack of an accurate screening test. Early detection is recommended for young males with a history of undescended testis (even if surgically corrected) or testicular atrophy, but not routine mass screening (USPSTF, 1989).

Cervical cancer. Screening is not recommended as a priority for well adolescents; it should be part of clinical care for those with repeated STD infections. Higher priority should be placed on screening those at higher risk, especially older women. Public health measures to promote the reduction of risk factors among young women (prevention of sexually transmitted diseases, family planning, smoking prevention) should have high priority (see page 131).

- **Haemoglobinopathies including sickle-cell trait**

Recommendation on use of screening. Not recommended as a priority unless universal coverage with well developed health services has been achieved. The homozygous condition would have become evident before adolescence. The screening of children and adolescents for haemoglobin-opathies aims to detect the carrier state with the hope that counselling will reduce the likelihood of two carriers having children. Counselling requires extensive training and skill, and there is no evidence of its effectiveness in preventing disease; thus, genetic screening for the carrier state should have relatively low priority in a primary health care context (see page 83).

● Rheumatic heart disease

Why. To identify those needing prophylaxis with antibiotics to prevent further damage through reinfection.

Who. All school-age children and adolescents in high-prevalence areas.

How. Auscultation of the heart with a stethoscope; requires examination by trained health professional. Will be possible only where all children can be examined by trained personnel (Finau & Taylor, 1988). Many false positives are recorded on clinical examination, and definitive diagnosis (echocardiography) and long-term penicillin prophylaxis will be too expensive in many developing countries.

When. At time of screening for immunizations.

Resource levels required. Medium or high for detection; medium or high for medical intervention (long-term antibiotic prophylaxis is expensive); very high if surgical intervention is needed.

Recommendation on use of screening. Not recommended as a priority where resources for definitive diagnosis and appropriate long-term antibiotic prophylaxis are not available for all persons found to be at risk. Efforts should focus on primary prevention through prompt and appropriate treatment for streptococcal infection.

CHAPTER 7

Screening of children and adults to prevent and control communicable diseases

This chapter discusses infectious diseases that endanger the health of the individual affected and sometimes others in the community. Because this material is generally relevant for all age groups, it was thought most convenient to present this as a separate chapter. Prevention and control of communicable diseases should be integral components of comprehensive primary health care programmes for each general age group, and should not be organized into separate vertical programmes focused on specific diseases.

General comments on screening for communicable diseases

In general, in dealing with highly prevalent communicable diseases that are a significant public health problem, the screening of asymptomatic persons will play a limited role and should be primarily an adjunct to other measures. Emphasis should be placed on primary prevention (often requiring environmental measures) and on public education regarding both primary prevention (preventing exposure) and the detection of early signs and symptoms with self-referral to services. A few specific examples are mentioned below. Acceptable, accessible services need to be provided for those at risk and those with symptoms. Targeted outreach and case-finding by health workers, especially for high-risk population groups unlikely to practise self-referral, may be needed to supplement the self-referral of an informed and motivated public. Case-finding may be neighbourhood-based (door-to-door or in market-places or other public places), workplace-based, or "opportunistic" (carried out in the course of delivering care sought for other purposes). Such case-finding efforts come under the heading of early detection of problems rather than screening.

Experience has shown that, for many important communicable diseases, primary care workers can be trained in early detection of relevant symptoms and signs; definitive diagnosis and treatment may require referral to facilities with additional resources. Wherever indigenous healers provide a substantial amount of care, both they and orthodox providers of care need to be trained in early detection.

Screening, early detection, and treatment for infectious diseases should be organized in a manner that is as convenient as possible for the population at risk and as efficient as possible. This implies maximum integration with other health services, including maternal and child health services (which in turn include services for reproductive health and family planning), and workplace-based health services. The integration of services into existing primary health

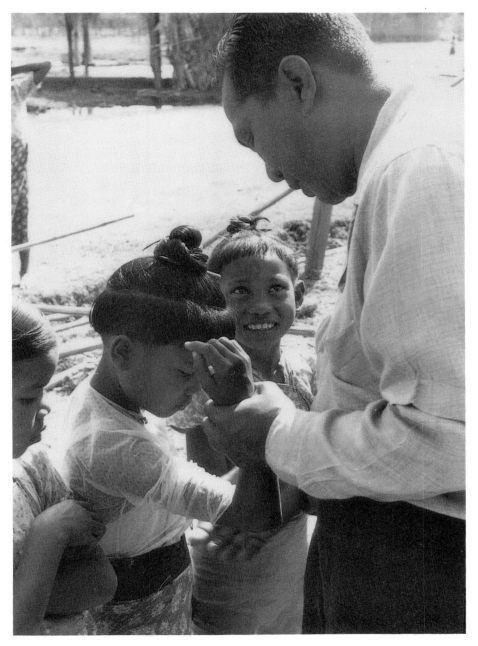

School-based early detection of leprosy in Myanmar.   (E. Scheidegger/WHO/6213A)

care programmes tends to increase the efficiency and effectiveness of short-term efforts to control infectious diseases, and at the same time helps strengthen permanent services. Under certain circumstances, e.g., during epidemics, it may be necessary to conduct special disease-specific campaigns for screening and treatment. Any proposal to implement a separate disease-specific screening effort outside the structure of the existing health services will require careful justification. Opportunities for coordination and integration with existing services should be actively pursued. For example, an emergency screening effort focused on HIV infection provides an opportunity to contribute to activities for the promotion of reproductive health, and the prevention of sexually transmitted diseases, in general. These opportunities should not be wasted. Efforts to prevent sexually transmitted diseases should be integrated with family planning methods.

There is an extensive literature on screening for communicable diseases in developing countries, with numerous examples of the successful use of primary care workers for screening in the community (neighbourhood, market, school, workplace, or peripheral health post), sometimes with referral to peripheral health posts or health centres for definitive diagnosis and treatment, and sometimes with treatment provided in the community by the primary care workers. We give below a few examples and make general comments about screening for communicable diseases; references are cited that are especially relevant to conditions in developing countries.

● Sexually transmitted diseases (STDs) other than HIV infection

Why. Early identification of most STDs other than HIV infection is of proven effectiveness in reducing morbidity and is thought to reduce further spread. Many STDs are asymptomatic until serious health damage has occurred and are also highly contagious, even when asymptomatic. STDs other than HIV infection and hepatitis B are generally curable with relatively simple treatments when detected opportunely.

Who and when. Regular screening of high-risk groups. Intervals between screening will depend on local resources and the education and motivation of the population at risk. Groups generally at high risk include heterosexuals with a number of partners or whose partners have a number of partners, homosexual or bisexual men, and prostitutes. In some areas, the criteria for high risk may be broader (see earlier recommendations for screening pregnant women and adolescents for STDs, pages 66–69 and 103–104 respectively).

How and where. Definitive diagnosis of STDs requires laboratory facilities and thus, even if primary care workers can be trained to take specimens, involves the use of technically trained personnel. While screening may be carried out at a peripheral health post, the processing of specimens will involve at least the resources of a health centre with a laboratory, and potentially the resources of a district laboratory. Communication systems are needed for sending specimens, ensuring timely delivery of results, notification of patients, and appropriate treatment and follow-up, with preservation of confidentiality throughout.

The presence of one STD generally indicates the need to consider others that are prevalent in the area. *Chlamydia trachomatis* infection has become more prevalent than gonorrhoea in many areas. Although cheaper antibody-based methods have recently been developed for chlamydia screening (Trachtenberg et al., 1988), the expense of accurate chlamydia screening may necessitate, in most places, giving presumptive treatment for chlamydia to persons with culture-proven gonorrhoea or relevant physical signs or symptoms or history (USPSTF, 1989).

Hepatitis B can be sexually transmitted and carriers may be asymptomatic. Homosexual and bisexual men, the female partners of bisexual men, prostitutes, users of intravenous drugs, and people who have received injections in unhygienic conditions are at risk. Unlike most other STDs, hepatitis B is not curable. The goal of screening would therefore be to reduce the likelihood of transmission; there is no evidence of the effectiveness of such an approach, compared with efforts to promote safe sexual practice.

Resource levels required. Low (enquiries regarding symptoms or risk factors) or medium to high (laboratory testing) for detection; low or medium for treatment of bacterial infections (antibiotics) and promotion of safe sex to prevent spread of disease and reinfection.

Recommendation on use of screening/early detection. Recommended to screen high-risk groups and pregnant women, confidentially and with informed consent. Early detection through "opportunistic" screening (for symptoms, exposure, or risk of exposure) is recommended, as is education for self-referral on the basis of potential exposure. Screening should be seen as an adjunct to other preventive activities, including public education on the prevention of STDs, the promotion of safe sexual practices, and the encouragement of self-referral for signs or symptoms of STDs or possible exposure to them. Services for screening, diagnosis, and treatment need to be confidential and readily accessible with special attention to the needs and preferences of the groups at highest risk.

● HIV infection

See discussion of HIV testing in prenatal health care, page 67. The same general issues apply in the non-pregnant population, except that the rationale for screening is more limited, since the issues of deciding whether to carry a pregnancy to term or whether to breast-feed are not involved. The primary rationale for screening the asymptomatic non-pregnant population at elevated risk (see page 68) is either to provide reassurance or to assist HIV-infected individuals in planning their lives. Even with a negative screening test result, however, reassurance can only be limited in view of the delay between infection and seroconversion. Community-wide education and the promotion of safe sexual practices are likely to have a far greater impact on HIV infection than a large-scale screening effort. Thus, our recommendation on HIV screening is uncertain at this time. Emphasis should be placed on primary prevention. If testing is done, resources need to be in place for skilled pre- and post-test counselling and social services for those found to be positive.

● Malaria

Screening of asymptomatic non-pregnant persons is not recommended as a priority in most situations. Epidemics and certain endemic situations may require mass screening of entire populations, including asymptomatic persons, to reduce continuous transmission (Krishnamoorthy et al., 1985). Screening will be only an adjunct to measures for environmental control and to ensuring that there are accessible services for the early detection of symptomatic persons, together with public education regarding signs and symptoms. The use of primary care workers in malaria screening and treatment is well established. The traditional approach has been to set up separate vertical malaria control programmes. Attempts to integrate malaria control activities within a broad primary health care strategy should be encouraged (WHO, 1993a,b). For example, malaria screening might be combined with screening and promotional activities relating to other important conditions affecting the population at risk for malaria, including not only other infectious diseases but also reproductive health problems and noncommunicable diseases.

● Tuberculosis

Screening of asymptomatic persons is not recommended where BCG vaccination is the norm. Emphasis should be on primary prevention through good housing and nutrition, along with early detection of persons with symptoms and treatment of household contacts of proven cases.

The tuberculin skin test can be used for screening in areas where BCG is not given, but it is difficult to interpret where BCG vaccination is common. Mass screening of asymptomatic persons with X-rays or sputum examinations is expensive and unproductive even in areas of relatively high prevalence (Aluoch et al., 1984; Gottridge et al., 1989; Kan, 1981; Krivinka et al., 1974; Stewart, 1966). Mass miniature X-ray screening may be an option where prevalence is particularly high and low-cost radiography widely available, but such screening may be of low specificity (Teklu & Kassegn, 1982). The risks of radiation exposure need to be considered, even with mass miniature techniques (Mustafi & Kouris, 1985). A paper published in 1978 concluded that case-finding by sputum microscopy performed by auxiliaries was "most suitable for Nepal", given the shortage of X-ray facilities and trained personnel and the low yield from mobile mass miniature radiography in other developing countries (Peresra, 1978).

A rational strategy may involve all of the following: measures to improve the general standard of living, including nutrition and housing conditions; BCG prophylaxis of newborn infants (with revaccination of schoolchildren found negative on tuberculin testing) (Kan, 1981); awareness that BCG vaccination does not confer 100% protection (Rai et al., 1987); "opportunistic" screening by the general medical services with referral for chest X-ray and sputum examination of those with persistent productive cough (Krivinka et al., 1974; Gatner & Burkhardt, 1980; PAHO, 1986); public education to encourage self-referral for symptoms, in places where the population has access to health services. A publication on tuberculosis control from the Pan American Health Organization calls attention to the fact that "opportunistic" screening efforts need to involve indigenous healers as well as those working in the mainstream health care system (PAHO, 1986).

● Leprosy, leishmaniasis, filariasis, and other endemic diseases with skin manifestations.

Screening of asymptomatic persons is generally not recommended. Follow-up of case contacts is recommended, as with any highly communicable disease. Mass screening is expensive. In endemic areas, it is more rational to use targeted case-finding by trained primary care workers who have regular contact with the population at risk, together with public education to promote self-referral for early detection of characteristic skin lesions (Ganapati et al., 1984), and the provision of accessible and acceptable general medical services for the population at risk. Skin manifestations are easily identifiable by primary care workers, and by an educated public in endemic regions. Ganapati et al. (1984) cite two earlier studies from rural areas in India to support their point that mass screening may add very little to the case detection achieved by other methods such as mass public health education. In settings with access to fairly high-technology laboratory resources, it may be an option to screen high-risk groups, such as the relatives of leprosy patients, with enzyme-linked immunosorbent assay techniques to detect subclinical disease (Britton et al., 1987). "Opportunistic" screening efforts need to involve indigenous healers as well as orthodox care providers.

● Schistosomiasis

Screening of asymptomatic persons is not recommended. As with many endemic parasitic diseases, opportune treatment will not be effective in the long term, without primary prevention (environmental control) to prevent repeated re-exposure. Screening should be seen as an adjunct to environmental control and education of the public to minimize exposure and to promote self-referral for gross haematuria (early detection). In many cases, the population will not have the option of avoiding exposure, for economic reasons; broad environmental control measures will almost always be required. Enquiry regarding history of haematuria has been used as an initial screen in adults, although gross inspection of urine is more accurate, especially in children (see page 107), followed by testing of urine for blood with reagent strips in the case of those found positive on initial screening (Mott et al., 1985).

• Onchocerciasis and trachoma

Screening of asymptomatic persons is not recommended. Early detection of signs and symptoms is recommended. In 1976, a WHO report on onchocerciasis recommended vector control rather than screening for this prevalent cause of blindness (WHO, 1976). A study in Sierra Leone has described a successful trial of school-based screening for onchocerciasis by an ophthalmologist; however, this would not be feasible in most developing countries (Stilma et al., 1983). Primary prevention and early detection of persons with symptoms are also the strategies recommended in a publication on the prevention of blindness issued by WHO in 1984 (WHO, 1984b). Where services are accessible, teaching the public to practise self-referral for symptoms (early detection) is a useful adjunct to primary prevention in endemic areas.

CHAPTER 8

Screening in the health care of adults

General comments

Routine mass screening of pregnant women and newborn infants, and of infants and children on the basis of the immunization schedule, has an important place in strategies for disease prevention and health promotion. Early detection of risks to mothers and children, with effective intervention, can be expected to make a substantial contribution to the overall improvement of a population's health in the long run. Routine mass screening of adults, however, has a more limited place in a primary health care system, for several reasons.

In the first place, pregnant women and young children are those most liable to suffer severe adverse effects in the absence of early detection and care for many relatively common conditions. Furthermore, there are highly effective ways of dealing with many of the most prevalent health problems of mothers and children at relatively low cost, for example, the identification and treatment of asymptomatic urinary tract infection or anaemia in pregnancy, the immunization of children, and detection of amblyopia or strabismus in young children. In addition, the routine minimum care of mothers and children, including immunization of infants and young children, entails periodic contact between the entire target population and health personnel. This creates a situation in which screening fits within and strengthens services designed for universal coverage and permits a more rational and equitable distribution of resources to those at highest risk within the population as a whole.

A rational approach to the screening of adults, on the other hand, more often involves the targeting of subgroups at particular risk. Furthermore, where universal coverage with basic health services has not been achieved, those adults who take advantage of preventive programmes for asymptomatic conditions tend to be better educated than the rest of the population and thus more aware of the value of preventive services. Where resources are extremely limited and significant proportions of the population do not have ready access to basic health services, adults seeking medical care for either acute or chronic illness also tend to be those with greater access to services than the rest (e.g., urban rather than rural dwellers). By contrast, in places that are relatively rich in resources and where virtually universal coverage with basic health services has been achieved, comprehensive health promotion services for adults, including periodic general health assessments integrated with counselling and health education, may make a genuine contribution to health promotion and disease prevention (Tatara et al., 1991).

Special attention must be given to ensuring appropriate targeting of screening to adult subpopulations at particular risk. The screening of populations at low risk for a given condition yields many false positive results, leading to the expense of definitive diagnosis, unnecessary anxiety, and the potential "labelling" of many people as "diseased". Especially where the appropriate treatment for a condition requires a relatively high level of technology and expense, the screening of low-risk populations who already have easy access to care will result in their increased demand for investment by the health system in a higher level of technology. This investment may be made at the expense of ensuring universal coverage of the population by more basic, less technologically complex services, which would have led to a greater improvement in health status for the population as a whole. The untargeted screening of adults – performed either as the opportunity occurs (i.e., when people attend clinical services for other reasons) or as part of specific screening operations – can thus divert resources away from those at highest risk towards a relatively small group of persons already receiving health care services.

The screening of those adults who are likely to be at highest risk can make possible the allocation of the available resources to those most in need and most likely to benefit from them. However, screening should not be used as a substitute for other, more effective preventive measures. Public education aimed at encouraging health promotion and self-referral for the early detection of important problems should be a fundamental component of any strategy for adult health. Such education should not be confined to adults, but should be part of a lifelong process beginning at school (Burenkov & Glasunov, 1982).

In addition to opportunities for screening adults through maternal and child health services, services at places of work and at marketplaces may be among the most promising ways of reaching adults, other than the elderly, with preventive and promotional activities. The workplace offers an opportunity for education, promotion, and follow-up. Offering adult screening services through maternal and child health programmes and workplace- and marketplace-based programmes is a means of striving for equity in resource allocation and improving access to care. Reaching elderly people with preventive services may require other approaches, especially to reach those who are socially isolated and housebound.

We have selected several noninfectious conditions or groups of conditions occurring in adults for which screening has been widely used, or for which targeted screening may have an important place within a primary health care strategy. As in previous chapters, we have not covered all conditions; nor have we covered any single condition in detail, although some topics (e.g., screening for cancer of the uterine cervix) are discussed at some length because they are good illustrations of important general principles. This chapter discusses the possible use of screening within a preventive strategy for the following groups of health problems or risk factors in adults: dental or periodontal disease; risk of unintended or high-risk pregnancy (also covered in Chapter 5, page 73, and in Chapter 6, page 104); psychosocial problems, including domestic violence and alcohol or drug abuse; problems of functional status in the elderly; cataracts

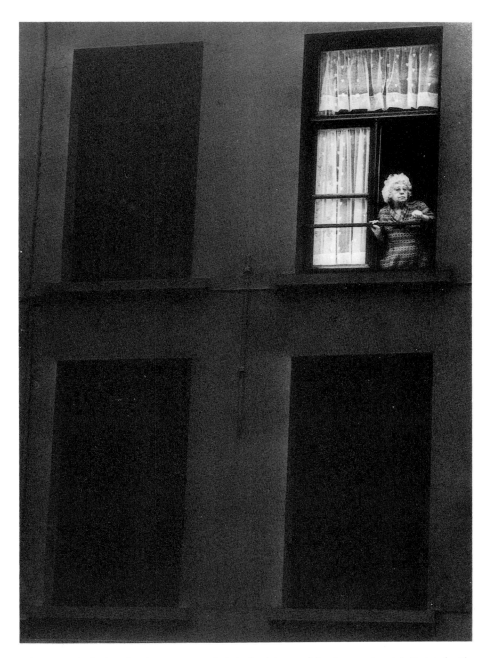

The social isolation that has accompanied the health transition is a major risk factor for the elderly.   (Zafar/WHO/21601)

and refractive errors; glaucoma; occupational hazards (covered only briefly, as another WHO publication deals with the subject (WHO, 1986a)); risk of cardiovascular and cerebrovascular disease (and vascular complications of diabetes mellitus); and cancer.

The reader will note that, throughout this section, but especially in the text dealing with cardiovascular and cancer risks, the US Preventive Services Task Force (USPSTF) is frequently cited. This is because theirs is the most recent and thorough review of the subjects at issue. Although it is based on conditions in the USA, much of this review appears highly relevant for developing countries. The Task Force has demonstrated that there is no scientific basis for performing many of the screening procedures to which the general adult population in some developed countries is routinely subjected. For example, the following are among the conditions for which the value of untargeted mass screening of the general population is not supported by the evidence: glaucoma (Gottlieb et al., 1983; Eddy et al., 1983); colorectal cancer; lung cancer; abnormalities indicated by electrocardiogram, chest X-ray, complete blood count, urinalysis, or blood chemistry for asymptomatic persons; and elevated blood sugar in the absence of clinical suspicion of diabetes mellitus (USPSTF, 1989; CTF, 1979; Eliakim et al., 1988). The prevalence of many of the noncommunicable diseases for which screening has been widely used is generally higher in the USA than in developing countries and resources are clearly more limited in the latter. The findings of the USPSTF recommending against screening for many noncommunicable diseases should thus be of significant value for policy-makers in developing countries.

General health problems

● Dental or periodontal disease

Why and how. Dental or periodontal disease is a significant cause of suffering and disability in adults in developing countries. Preventive efforts (hygiene, fluoridation) need to be targeted to the whole population from childhood on. Early detection in adults has, as its primary goals, pain control and preservation of function. Unpublished reports indicate that it is possible to train primary care workers to recognize dental or periodontal disease which can be treated at the local or district level with limited resources (MH LeClercq, personal communication, 1989; A Yashin, personal communication, 1987). In areas where there is a high prevalence of oral cancer, it appears rational to integrate dental and periodontal screening with oral cancer screening.

Resource levels required. Low for screening; medium for definitive diagnosis and treatment.

Recommendation on use of screening. Recommended to screen all adults; frequency of screening needs to be determined by local resources. Primary prevention from childhood on should also be a high priority.

● **Risk of unintended or high-risk pregnancy**

Why. To refer for family planning services.

Who. All women and men of reproductive age should ideally be screened, as the opportunity arises, within maternal and child health programmes and health services for adults. In areas where such an approach would be culturally acceptable, consider "opportunistic" screening of all adults of reproductive age receiving medical care for other reasons.

How. Screen by enquiry in a confidential setting. Can be done by primary care workers with training in how to maintain confidentiality. The home-based maternal record, which contains a section for information on intervals between pregnancies, as well as covering several pregnancies, constitutes an excellent means of reminding health workers to enquire about the need for family planning.

When. As the opportunity arises within maternal and child health programmes and general medical care.

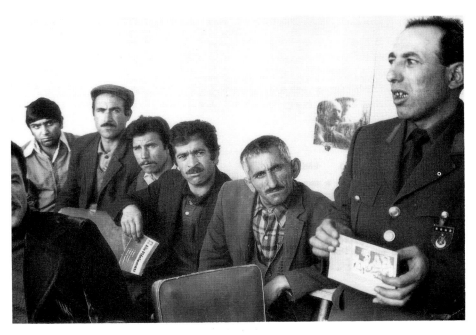

The reduction of unintended or high-risk pregnancies will depend primarily on continuous mass public education and on the availability of safe, effective, and acceptable family planning services; here a health worker talks about family planning to men in a pub in Turkey. (J. Mohr/WHO/16791)

Resource levels required. Low for detection; intervention may require resource levels that are low (education regarding family planning, emphasizing use of barrier methods), medium (prescription of oral contraceptives or diaphragm, vasectomy), or high (tubal ligation).

Recommendation on use of screening. "Opportunistic" screening and early detection of problems are recommended but are likely to play a very limited role in reducing the risk. The reduction of unintended or high-risk pregnancies will depend primarily on continuous mass public education reaching men as well as women, and on the availability of safe, effective, and acceptable family planning services.

● Psychosocial problems, including problems of mental health, alcohol and drug abuse, and domestic violence

"Patients whose mental disorders are presented somatically are frequent users of medical services and form a substantial proportion of all patients seen in developing countries. There is evidence that provision of psychiatric care reduces subsequent use of medical services, so there would appear to be economic as well as humanitarian reasons for improving the detection and treatment of mental disorders in medical settings" (Hamburg, 1989). On the other hand, according to the USPSTF (1989), "it has not been demonstrated in a controlled setting that the detection and treatment of alcohol or other drug abuse through screening of asymptomatic persons can produce a better outcome than conventional treatment after signs and symptoms become apparent ... However ... some studies support the efficacy of counselling once the signs or symptoms of problem drinking ... are detected."

Screening for psychological problems may be desirable under certain circumstances, for example, where it is suspected that such problems account for a high proportion of medical service use without benefit, or after the occurrence of a major disaster (Lima et al., 1987). The literature contains references to apparently successful experiments in which primary care workers with little formal education and limited training conducted screening with standardized instruments designed for use in developing countries, including the rural areas (Sen et al., 1987; Khare et al., 1988).

Why and how. Mental health problems, alcohol and drug abuse, and domestic violence are important public health problems in whose management routine screening would appear not to have a significant place. Where referral resources exist, health workers should be trained to recognize psychosocial problems and make appropriate referrals. Studies show a low pick-up rate of mental disorders by providers not performing formal screening. Formal self-report questionnaires may have limited validity for screening a general population (Hoeper et al., 1984; Oduwole & Ogunyemi, 1989).

Resource levels required. Low for screening by primary care worker; low or medium for definitive diagnosis; low, medium, or high for intervention by specialized counselling personnel.

Recommendation on use of screening/early detection. Uncertain recommendation on "opportunistic" screening because of the lack of firm evidence of the effectiveness of intervention when the person affected does not seek help. Early detection of household risks for children recommended. The primary prevention of psychosocial problems should be emphasized.

Research priority. A very high priority should be placed on research to develop effective primary prevention, early detection, and treatment methods at the primary care level.

● Problems of functional status in the elderly

Why. Increased life expectancy has made the health of the elderly an issue of concern in most countries. Changes in society also make the social isolation of the elderly a problem not restricted to the industrialized world. The elderly are vulnerable, and it should be possible to design appropriate ways of promoting an optimum quality of life for the elderly in a primary health care context. Screening for cataracts, a common and treatable cause of blindness in the elderly, is addressed below.

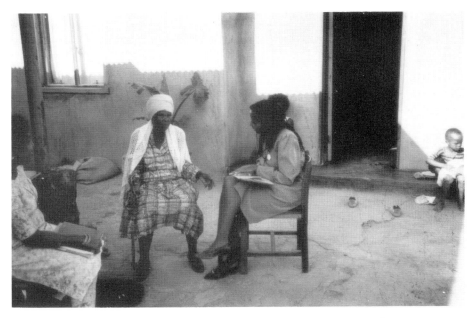

A home visit to an elderly woman combines assessment and support services.

How. A recent essay aimed at general practitioners in the United Kingdom urges "that screening [of the elderly] should be oriented to the patient's functioning and not to disease" (Freer, 1990). Periodic assessment is recommended, including assessment of mobility, social and mental functioning, hearing, vision, and continence, and a review of medication; the author also recommends an annual home visit. The USPSTF (1989) has stressed assessment of functional status as an essential component of preventive care for the elderly.

It appears worth while to train primary care workers to make routine functional assessments of elderly persons in the community, especially those with precarious social support. The goal would not be to detect disease but to detect functional limitations that could be relieved with simple measures within the reach of local resources and to promote maximal functional status (WHO, 1989b). Simple multidimensional assessment tools and interventions that could be used by primary care workers need to be developed and validated (Cooper & Bickel, 1984; Fillenbaum, 1985; Beers et al., 1991).

Resource levels required. Low for screening by primary care worker; low or medium for definitive diagnosis and for intervention, including simple supportive social interventions.

Recommendation on use of screening. Screening of the elderly for functional status is recommended as a priority, along with early detection of diminished mental or physical function.

Research priority. Developing simple but accurate assessment tools that can be used by primary care workers, together with ways of training primary care workers to deal effectively with the risks detected (tertiary prevention).

● Cataracts and refractive errors

Why. Cataracts are a leading cause of preventable blindness in the elderly. New methods of cataract surgery do not require a hospital stay. Many elderly people consider limited visual acuity a normal part of the aging process and thus not symptomatic of any disease, despite significant reversible disability.

Who. Elderly people.

How. Screening by enquiry and observation, ideally making use of a visual chart or appropriate pictorial substitute.

When. Frequency uncertain.

Resource levels required. Low for initial screening by enquiry or simple assessment of acuity, which can be done by trained primary care workers (Venkataswamy, 1972); medium for optometric examination; high for cataract extraction or corrective lenses, but there are ways in which this secondary-level medical care can be provided at relatively low cost in developing countries (WHO, 1984b).

Recommendation on use of screening/early detection. Screening/early detection is recommended in the elderly, not only as the opportunity presents itself but as part of routine periodic population-wide assessments of functional status, at intervals that will depend on local resources. Because many elderly people and those looking after them do not consider blindness as pathological, we have categorized the early detection of this problem as an example of screening. Early detection is recommended in other age groups through provision of services and education of the public to promote self-referral. People with diabetes mellitus should be under special surveillance for proliferative retinopathy, another common treatable cause of blindness in adults.

● Glaucoma

Why. Glaucoma is an important cause of irreversible blindness; effective treatment exists for high levels of intraocular pressure, but this condition is rare in the general population under the age of 65. No clear evidence exists that early intervention for moderately increased levels of intraocular pressure in asymptomatic persons leads to improved outcome (WHO, 1984b; USPSTF, 1989).

How and resource levels required. Screening and definitive diagnosis by means of tonometry, ophthalmoscopy, and perimetry (all requiring medium or high resource levels); screening by non-specialists is of uncertain efficacy. Intervention: medium (medication to reduce intraocular pressure) or high (surgery).

Recommendation on use of screening. Screening of the general population is not recommended as a priority. Persons at special risk should be under special surveillance (Eddy et al., 1983; Gottlieb et al., 1983; USPSTF, 1989). The elderly should be screened for visual problems; those with problems should receive diagnostic testing.

● Occupational hazards

Recommendation on use of screening. Uncertain recommendation on routine screening of general population regarding occupational exposures. "Opportunistic" screening may be reasonable, especially in areas where it is known that the population is exposed to occupational hazards. The benefit of questioning individuals during routine health care is uncertain. It appears reasonable to ask about potential occupational hazards when completing an adult's health history; however, this may not lead to effective action. The most rational strategy is one that emphasizes primary prevention and routine monitoring of workplaces.

Workers in high-risk occupations should be screened for relevant immunization status on starting employment. There should be routine surveillance of workplaces to detect and minimize hazards. This, along with training workers and ensuring that they are properly equipped, should be at the centre of a preventive strategy, with screening only an adjunct. Certain persons may be more vulnerable to hazards than others, for biological or psychosocial reasons. Workers exposed to certain risks may need periodic surveillance to permit early detection of adverse effects, followed, where indicated, by reassignment to less hazardous tasks. For further information on occupational health screening, the reader is referred to two previous WHO publications (WHO, 1975, 1986a).

Cardiovascular and cerebrovascular diseases

Cardiovascular and cerebrovascular diseases are now among the most frequent causes of morbidity and premature mortality in many developing countries. Screening has a limited role in strategies aimed at reducing the risks of cardiovascular and cerebrovascular disease. The literature on this subject has been carefully reviewed by the Canadian and US task forces; the work of the US Preventive Services Task Force (USPSTF, 1989) is the most recent and involved consultation with key members of the Canadian Task Force. The conclusions of the USPSTF are summarized here, as a point of departure for recommendations focusing on the special needs of developing countries.

Given the greater prevalence of cardiovascular and cerebrovascular diseases in industrialized countries, it is of relevance to policy-makers in developing countries that the USPSTF recommended against routine electrocardiography (ECG), chest X-rays, lipid profile testing (including cholesterol and triglyceride screening), and auscultation for carotid bruits, as mass screening techniques. They emphasized regular counselling of patients by physicians and other health care providers on ways of reducing cardiovascular risks (stopping smoking, reducing alcohol intake, diet, exercise). They recommended routine screening (by enquiry) combined with counselling of all adults aged 19–64 every 1–3 years, and of those aged 65 and over annually, for dietary risks, physical activity, and tobacco, alcohol, and drug use.

● Risks associated with diet, exercise, or substance use, including tobacco

Why. "Opportunistic" screening has been recommended to health care providers in North America, so that patients whose behaviour is damaging to their health can be counselled. Tobacco, alcohol, high-salt diet, and sedentary habits are major risk factors for hypertension and ischaemic heart disease, which are now important causes of suffering and premature mortality in most developing countries. It appears that advice from a sympathetic health care provider can help individuals change their behaviour, leading to health-promoting changes; such advice may be especially effective when the care provider is well known to the patient.

Who. All adults.

How and when. Enquiry (verbal; questionnaires with literate population). Optimal frequency of screening and counselling is not established.

Resource levels required. Low for detection (enquiry); low or medium for intervention (counselling and referral to appropriate support services).

Recommendation on use of screening. Not recommended. Emphasis should be on primary prevention and making treatment available for persons who wish to change their habits. The approach must be country-specific.

Research priority. Development of effective methods of primary prevention and treatment for persons seeking help in giving up health-damaging behaviour.

● High blood pressure

The USPSTF has recommended routine blood pressure screening of all adults every 1–3 years from ages 19 to 64, and annually from the age of 65 on, citing firm evidence of an association between early treatment of adults with mild, moderate, or malignant hypertension and a reduction in coronary artery disease and mortality from stroke. Benefits are greatest with early treatment of those whose blood pressure is highest. However, the US Task Force's discussion distinguished between efficacy of treatment (in careful clinical trials) and its effectiveness in actual practice. They noted the problems often encountered with medication, including high cost and frequent difficulty in getting patients to take it because of inconvenience of administration and unpleasant side-effects, as well as with nonpharmacological recommendations for weight reduction, salt restriction, increased physical activity, and decreased alcohol intake. Patient compliance with recommendations to change behaviour is often poor; furthermore, some people with hypertension are not sensitive to salt.

Even more difficult questions arise when blood pressure screening is considered from the standpoint of a developing country. High blood pressure may be especially prevalent in many nations with severe limitations on health spending. The minimum annual cost per person treated with the least expensive anti-hypertension drugs is estimated at US $54.00, not including the cost of monitoring or follow-up consultations. With a 10% prevalence of hypertension among adults in several African nations (Oviasu & Okupa, 1980), the pharmacological treatment of all people with high blood pressure could consume more than the annual health budget for the entire country (I Gyárfás, personal communication, 1989).

Since those who enjoy the greatest benefit in reduced mortality are those with the highest blood pressure levels before treatment, it may be necessary in certain places, in view of limited resources, to use a higher threshold for the blood-pressure reading when pharmacological treatment is instituted. Those identified as having hypertension but under the threshold for pharmacological therapy could be targeted for intensified action through the nonpharmacological reduction of risk factors. Appropriate screening would be a way of ensuring that scarce resources are allocated to those in greatest need. A decision to undertake mass blood-pressure screening needs to be based on prior calculations of the cost not only of screening, but of long-term treatment, and a consideration of the implications for the health budget as a whole.

Trained primary care workers can screen for high blood pressure. It is important to note, however, that blood pressure screening with appropriate treatment of adults attending general medical services, without efforts to screen those sections of the population not using existing services, will result in an increased concentration of resources on those who already benefit most. In places where virtually universal coverage has been achieved, this might not be a problem, and could in fact be the most efficient approach (Bryers & Hawthorne, 1978). Where universal coverage with basic services has not yet been achieved, however, a decision regarding introducing blood pressure screening among nonpregnant adults should be made in full awareness of the implications and with careful consideration of alternatives.

The difficulties of long-term follow-up of hypertension in non-elderly adults might be addressed particularly effectively in a workplace setting, where promotional efforts could be reinforced and inconvenience would be minimized. Workplace-based programmes could offer an opportunity for screening for other risks as well as hypertension, and for long-term follow-up with treatment (A Griffiths et al., unpublished data, 1984). On the other hand, such an effort could require a considerable investment in initial and long-term support, which may not be feasible in certain places.

Mass community-based screening (e.g., blood-pressure screening in markets and other public places) has been used to increase public awareness of the problem and promote self-referral for care to existing health services (Flancbaum et al., 1978; Silverberg et al., 1974). Such an approach can be effective only if there are acceptable, accessible services with good follow-up capability. The capacity of existing services to respond adequately to the additional demand created by this kind of outreach needs to be carefully calculated in advance. An evaluation of a population survey for hypertension and diabetes in Fiji in 1980 (Tuomilehto et al., 1987) concluded that "simple population screening for hypertension and diabetes may result in an extra work load and limit the available health care resources so that the overall outcome is not satisfactory".

Screening and medical treatment should be accompanied by broad public health action to reduce risk factors, e.g., legislation to ban tobacco advertising and prohibit the sale of tobacco products to minors, and public education aimed at preventing smoking and reducing dietary intake of salt and animal fats. Effective health education is difficult to carry out and requires sensitivity to local cultural and socioeconomic issues as well as an allocation of sufficient resources for development and implementation of programmes that will have an impact.

Resource levels required. Low for detection; medium technology for intervention but costly in the long term.

Recommendation on use of screening. Uncertain. Not recommended for general population when resources are insufficient to give long-term treatment and monitoring to all who have hypertension. Targeted screening of the groups at highest risk is recommended when resources are adequate for their long-term treatment. Emphasis should be on primary prevention (smoking cessation; promotion of healthy diet and exercise).

Research priorities. Cheaper treatment methods and effective community-wide strategies for primary prevention.

● Elevated blood cholesterol

The USPSTF (1989) recommended periodic screening of non-fasting total blood cholesterol of all adults, leaving the frequency to "clinical discretion". Evidence is especially strong of the benefit (in terms of reduced mortality from coronary artery disease) of early detection and treatment with cholesterol-lowering drugs for European and white American men aged 35–59 years and mostly middle-class, with very high serum cholesterol (> 255 mg/dl). However, questions remain about the applicability of the findings to other groups, including women, younger men, the elderly, other racial or socioeconomic groups, and persons whose cholesterol levels are not quite so high. The USPSTF stressed the importance of repeated measurements to confirm the diagnosis, a single reading being unreliable.

The high cost of repeated measurements of blood cholesterol plus long-term treatment with cholesterol-lowering drugs, combined with the uncertain implications of the findings in middle-aged European and white American men for populations in developing countries, suggests that screening for high cholesterol should not be a priority within a strategy for primary health care. The evidence appears clearer for screening and treating hypertension, which should thus have higher priority, along with measures to reduce other risk factors in the population as a whole, including smoking, obesity, excessive alcohol intake, and high dietary intake of salt and, possibly, animal fats (Browner et al., 1991). It would be rational to target screening to those with a family history of early coronary artery disease, rather than the general population.

Resource levels required. Medium technology for detection but costly because of need for repeated measurements; low or medium for intervention (diet counselling); medium for medication (expensive).

Recommendation on use of screening. Screening of the general adult population in the absence of specific risk factors is not recommended. Emphasis should be on primary prevention.

● Carotid bruits

Why. To identify people at risk of cerebrovascular accidents, for medical (anticoagulant) or surgical (carotid endarterectomy) intervention.

How. Auscultation (stethoscope) or Doppler ultrasound. Definitive diagnosis requires arteriography.

Resource levels required. Medium, high, or very high for detection. Very high for intervention with carotid endarterectomy.

Recommendation on use of screening. Screening of asymptomatic adults is not recommended. Accurate detection involves invasive tests that are expensive and have serious associated risks. Intervention is extremely expensive and of uncertain long-term benefit. A recent large clinical trial in the USA found no evidence "that vascular surgery prevents stroke in patients with asymptomatic . . . carotid stenosis" demonstrated on screening (Pierce, 1992). Emphasis should be on primary prevention through reduction of risk factors for cerebrovascular disease (smoking prevention or cessation, diet, exercise) in the community.

● **Elevated blood sugar** (diabetes mellitus; glucose intolerance)

Chronic hyperglycaemia can eventually lead to blindness, gangrene of the extremities, and renal failure as well as being a contributory factor to the risk of cardiovascular disease and stroke. There is still some controversy regarding the benefit of "tight control" of blood sugar in reducing microvascular and macrovascular complications, and there is inadequate evidence that early detection and treatment improve the outcome in asymptomatic persons. There is no convenient, inexpensive, and accurate screening test: urine glucose testing is nonsensitive and nonspecific; a random blood glucose measurement is insufficiently sensitive or specific; fasting blood glucose measurement is more accurate but inconvenient and limited in sensitivity; postprandial testing is not convenient; the 75-g oral glucose tolerance test is most accurate, but is inconvenient and very costly (oral glucose load and numerous venepunctures at specified intervals) (USPSTF, 1989).

The most common form of diabetes is the adult-onset type (AODM). The major risk factors for AODM are obesity, family history, and history of gestational diabetes. While many persons with AODM require insulin or oral agents, the condition tends to be responsive to weight control.

For all these reasons, the USPSTF recommended against population-wide screening of asymptomatic non-pregnant persons for glucose intolerance. It recommended that all patients should be encouraged to control their weight and take healthy exercise and that the screening of adults who are markedly obese, have a family history of diabetes, or have a history of gestational diabetes should be considered (see comments on screening for gestational diabetes, page 70).

Within a primary health care strategy, the mass screening of asymptomatic adults for glucose intolerance does not appear to be justified (Tuomilehto et al., 1987). Public education to reduce the major risk factors for cardiovascular, cerebrovascular, and peripheral vascular disease (including tobacco use and obesity) would be a high priority. In addition, screening of high-risk groups may be an option where universal coverage with basic health services has been achieved and there is the infrastructure required for the identification and effective treatment of those at greatest risk.

Resource levels required. Medium for detection; medium for intervention (diet counselling, oral medications, insulin).

Recommendation on use of screening. Screening of asymptomatic persons for hyperglycaemia is not recommended.

Cancer

Under certain conditions, the targeted screening of groups of adults at increased risk of cervical, breast, and oral cancer is recommended as a tool for primary health care. The targeting criteria for those conditions are summarized below. Screening of pregnant women for hepatitis B surface antigen, combined with immunization of the newborn infants of antigen-positive mothers, has been effective in preventing primary liver cancer in some areas of high prevalence (WHO, 1983; Sun et al., 1986); where prevalence is particularly high, however, universal vaccination of newborns, without screening, may be more efficient. Screening of whole populations for colorectal cancer is not currently recommended as part of a primary health care strategy, owing to the lack of an accurate, acceptable, inexpensive screening technique (Winawer & Miller, 1987; Eliakim et al., 1988; USPSTF, 1989).

● Cervical cancer[1]

Why. Cervical cancer is the most common cancer in women in developing countries and is curable if detected early. Targeted screening for cervical cancer is highly recommended within a primary health care strategy when the capacity exists, preferably at the district level, for reaching the women at highest risk. Targeted screening and treatment should be combined with action for primary prevention through the provision of access to safe family planning methods, the prevention and control of STDs, and the prevention of smoking which is an important risk factor for cervical carcinoma. The women at highest risk are those over 35 years of age and those with STDs.

---

[1] The following are excellent general sources of information on experience with cervical cancer screening in developing countries: Abeyewickreme, 1989; Ayangade & Akinyemi, 1989; Engineer & Misra, 1987; Garud et al., 1983; Lunt, 1984; Luthra et al., 1988; Lynch et al., 1985; Pinotti et al., 1981; Sampaio Goes et al., 1981; Schneider & Meinhardt, 1984; Shrivastav et al., 1986; Tao et al., 1984; Yang et al., 1985.

Who, how, and when. WHO has developed recommendations for cervical cancer screening that are relevant to the needs of developing countries (WHO Meeting, 1986; Stanley et al., 1987; Stjernswärd et al., 1987). WHO Collaborating Centres have made important contributions in that area (Habbema, 1990). The following comments are a summary of those findings.

A phased-in approach is rational wherever shortage of resources makes it impossible to cover all women at risk with screening through Pap smears at suitable intervals. One of the key limiting factors in many countries will be the number of trained cytotechnicians or cytotechnologists available to read smears accurately. First, every women should have a Pap smear once between the ages of 35 and 40. "When more resources are available the frequency of screening should be increased to once every five or ten years for the age groups 35 to 55 years and, ideally, once every three years for women aged between 25 and 60 years" (WHO Meeting, 1986). It is worth noting that women over 65 who have been repeatedly found negative in previous Pap smears do not need further testing (USPSTF, 1989).

According to this phased-in approach, priority is given first to expanding the coverage of women in the age groups at highest risk and subsequently to increasingly frequent screening of those covered. The coverage of women aged 35 and over will require a special public education and outreach effort, because such people are generally not reached by maternal and child health services. Most of the population at risk could be missed if efforts are concentrated on antepartum and postpartum women, women bringing their children for well-child care, and women seeking help with family planning.

It is common practice in many countries to make Pap smear screening a routine component of care for women seen by family planning services. In places where the older population is not yet covered and only a limited number of Pap smears can be done, this practice should be reconsidered within the framework of the phased-in approach described above. The effectiveness of cervical cancer screening is more likely to be improved by extending testing to women who are not being screened and by improving the accuracy and follow-up of Pap smears than by frequent re-screening of the same women (USPSTF, 1989).

Coverage should not be expanded without a guaranteed infrastructure to ensure effective follow-up (timely return of results to the responsible care provider and to the patient), definitive diagnosis, and treatment. Treatment should be made available as close to home as possible, since some women, especially those with very young children, may refuse treatment that requires them to leave their families. The treatment offered should include curative treatment when possible; where cure is not possible, it should include effective palliative therapy to relieve pain.

The option of using visual examination instead of cytology as the initial screening technique has been suggested as worth exploring in places where resources are particularly scarce (Stjernswärd et al., 1987; Luthra et al.,

1988; Miller, 1992). Under this option, primary care workers or auxiliaries are trained to carry out a visual examination of the cervix, using a speculum and without taking a specimen for cytology. Cytology is performed only on those at highest risk because of their history, or those with a suspicious examination or with symptoms. This approach is known as "downstaging", i.e., the detection of disease in an early stage when still curable, by non-medical health workers. The phased-in approach, based on expanding coverage before increasing screening frequency, is used, and the public is educated to seek services. However, visual inspection would miss many cases of dysplasia (Garud et al., 1983; Yang et al., 1985; Engineer & Misra 1987). The assumption behind the downstaging approach using visual examination is that, in many cases, the natural history of cervical carcinoma is relatively slow, and there is thus considerable time between the appearance of a clinically detectable lesion and the development of incurable disease (Stjernswärd et al., 1987; Luthra et al., 1988). This is a promising approach that requires testing for effectiveness; it is intended for application where resources are severely limited, which may not be the case in all developing countries.

Pending results of studies of the use of visual examination of the cervix as the initial screening technique, another option is to use the system of priorities suggested by WHO studies, and maximize the use of trained paramedical workers to perform Pap smears (Sampaio Goes et al., 1981; Luthra et al., 1988). Alternative suggestions are that one cytological screening should be carried out for all women with parity greater than two, regardless of age (Shrivastav et al., 1986; Ayangade & Akinyemi, 1989) and that screening should be repeated every 5 years, especially for those with additional risk factors (smoking, prior dysplasia or malignancy, a sexually transmitted disease, a number of male partners, or a single male partner with a number of partners).

Another option, which is clearly preferable if resources permit, is to perform cytology once on all heterosexually active women aged 20–64, or with parity greater than two regardless of age, and to repeat the screening one year later to rule out false negatives. For women with two normal smears and no special risks, screening may be repeated every 5–10 years, with more frequent screening for those with additional risk factors.

Skilled technicians can be trained to do a first reading, with a pathologist reviewing equivocal or suspicious smears, and carrying out spot checks of random samples for quality control. All smears should be sent to a central laboratory so that the technician can have enough work to maintain a sufficiently high level of skill (J Stjernswärd, personal communication, 1989).

Screening and treatment need to be done in a manner consonant with cultural values. In most places, this will mean that screening should be done by women care providers. Attention needs to be paid to the issues of privacy and confidentiality; this may require a special effort during training and the organization of services and information systems, when primary care workers are involved and support of the community for follow-up action is sought.

At the time of screening there must already be a realistic plan in place for ensuring that information on the examination or test result gets back to the women screened, together with support for appropriate follow-up action. Such support may involve community organizations, as in a study in Lesotho, where village chiefs helped locate women with abnormal results who did not return for follow-up (Schneider & Meinhardt, 1984; Lynch et al., 1985) and encouraged them to receive care. The treatment plan needs to take into account transport difficulties, economic pressures, and social responsibilities, including child care, that may hinder appropriate follow-up, especially in rural areas.

Also at the time screening is initiated, facilities need to be available within or near the district, at least for carrying out conization for cancer *in situ* and localized cancer, and possibly for performing hysterectomy. Ideally, a facility for radiotherapy should be readily available. Resources should be allocated for medication to control pain for those with disseminated disease.

Resource levels required. Low or medium for screening by visual inspection, but the technique requires more validation; high for cervical cytology; low or medium for palliation of pain with medication; high for cone biopsy or other surgery or very high if radiation therapy required.

Recommendation on use of screening. Screening of high-risk women (aged 35–55, or with high parity, or with history of STD) with cervical cytology (Papanicolaou smear of cervical cells) is recommended as a priority. Recent studies suggest that, if it is not possible to carry out cytology for all women in the high-risk category, it is advisable to screen initially by visual inspection of the cervix and carry out cytological testing for suspicious findings. The recommendation is uncertain regarding cytological screening of low-risk groups. It is not recommended to carry out frequent cytological screening of low-risk groups before the high-risk population has been adequately covered. Emphasis should be placed on primary prevention through smoking cessation, family planning, and prevention and early detection of STDs.

Research priority. Validation of low-cost accurate methods of screening.

● Breast cancer in women[1]

Why. Cancer of the breast is the leading cause of cancer deaths in women in many developing countries, as well as in most developed countries. Early detection can significantly improve the chances of survival (Stanley et al., 1987) as well as quality of life, making far less radical therapy necessary.

---

[1] A recent review is by Miller (1991). Other useful papers on developing country experiences with breast cancer screening are by Fernandez et al. (1986), Persaud (1987), and Slater et al. (1981).

Current use of lumpectomy rather than mastectomy in many cases makes treatment more acceptable than in previous years.

Who and how. The USPSTF (1989) recommends annual clinical examination of the breasts in women aged 35 and older with a family history of premenopausal breast cancer in a first-degree relative, and of all women aged 40 and over. They recommend mammography every 1–2 years in the high-risk group, and every 1–2 years for all women aged 50–75. The Canadian Task Force recommended an annual clinical examination and mammography for all women between the ages of 50 and 59 and only an annual clinical examination for those aged 40 to 49 (CTF, 1986; Morrison, 1986). The WHO Collaborating Centre in the Netherlands supported recommendations that all women aged 50–70 in that country should be screened with mammography every two years, with mobile units providing examination in some areas (Habbema, 1990). There is still controversy in developed countries about the cost-effectiveness of mass mammography in various age groups (van der Maas et al., 1989). It is clear that mass mammography (estimated cost US $50–100 per mammogram) as an initial screen will be beyond the means of developing countries for the immediate future. Some alternative approaches are outlined below.

Screening for breast cancer should first be targeted to women aged 50 and over, with coverage of younger women being gradually phased in once older women are adequately covered (CTF, 1986; Morrison, 1986; Stanley et al., 1987; USPSTF, 1989). The best approach would be annual physical examination by a trained professional, together with mammography (Miller, 1989). Where mammography cannot be performed on all women over 50, frequent clinical examination by a trained professional, with mammography for suspected cases, may be the best option, though it is as yet an untested technique and one that is not highly sensitive or specific (Pavlov & Semiglazov, 1981).

Where mammography cannot be performed for all women at high risk, a worthwhile alternative may be public education to promote self-examination by all women over the age of 20, with more intensive screening, if possible, for women of 50 and over and those with a family history of breast cancer (Stanley et al., 1987). Large-scale prospective controlled studies of self-examination of breasts as an initial screening technique were initiated under the auspices of WHO in 1985 in what was then the USSR, and in 1989 in what was then the German Democratic Republic; preliminary reports indicate its feasibility (Semiglazov & Moissenko, 1987; WHO, 1989c) and early data on its effects are expected in the near future.

In 1990, Koroltchouk et al. stated "All three main elements — public education, early detection and locally available treatment — must be part of a breast cancer control program. These program elements can be delivered through existing health care infrastructures at almost any stage of development, given that there is a serious commitment of current resources. The use of perhaps nonoptimal but realistic available technology and the application of current knowledge would allow the extension of care to many patients who now die without diagnosis, treatment, and palliation."

Resource levels required. Low for screening by self-examination but the technique requires further validation, medium for clinical examination, high for mammography or biopsy; high for surgery and chemotherapy; very high for radiation therapy.

Recommendation on use of screening. Uncertain, owing to inadequate evidence on the accuracy of the available screening tests that would be affordable on a population-wide basis in developing countries. Routine mammography for women aged 50 or over appears to be quite accurate, but is beyond the resources of most developing countries at present; the capacity to perform it should have high priority as a goal for the future. Women should be made more aware of breast cancer and encouraged to practise self-referral for suspicious lumps or skin changes.

Research priority. Validation of low-cost, accurate methods of screening and early detection.

● **Oral cancer**

Why and how. Oral cancer accounts for approximately one-third of all cancers in Bangladesh, India, Pakistan, and Sri Lanka (WHO Meeting, 1984). It is thought to be especially prevalent in south-east Asian countries because of the widespread use of tobacco, especially mixed in as an ingredient of chewed betel quid (Warnakulasuriya et al., 1984). Like cervical cancer, oral cancer has a relatively long precancerous stage, which is treatable, so that early detection is particularly worth while. In a field study in Sri Lanka, 34 primary care workers, after a brief training course, screened 28 295 people in one year; the sensitivity and specificity of the screening were assessed as high. The main problem noted was a low rate of follow-up for the treatment of those with abnormalities, indicating a need to re-examine the organization of follow-up services (Warnakulasuriya et al., 1988); nevertheless, the results were considered to validate the approach to screening. A "look a friend in the mouth" campaign in areas of high prevalence to educate people to check each other for visible lesions and seek health services, appears promising; its effectiveness is being tested.

A primary health care approach would combine screening, early detection, and treatment with action for the primary prevention of oral and oropharyngeal cancer through legislation and education to control the production, distribution, advertising, and use of tobacco (Stanley & Stjernswärd, 1986).

Resource levels required. Low for screening by primary care workers; medium or high for definitive diagnosis and treatment.

Recommendation on use of screening. Screening for oral cancer is recommended in areas of high prevalence. Community-based approaches have been shown to be feasible; their effectiveness is being tested in a range of settings. Emphasis should be on primary prevention through efforts to prevent the use of tobacco products and other oral carcinogens (e.g., betel).

● Colorectal cancer

Screening of asymptomatic persons for colorectal cancer is not recommended as a priority at present. Many false positives and false negatives are yielded by affordable screening tests (Ahlquist et al., 1993) and evidence for the benefits of screening is inconclusive (USPSTF, 1989). While screening by sigmoidoscopy may be efficacious (Levin, 1992; Selby et al., 1992), it is expensive and of low acceptability in many cultures. Emphasis should be on primary prevention through a high-fibre diet.

Resource levels required. Medium for screening by testing for faecal occult blood or digital rectal examination, but results are inconclusive; high for sigmoidoscopy, radiological studies, and biopsy; high for surgery.

● Prostate cancer

Screening of asymptomatic men is not recommended as a priority at the present time. Many false positives are obtained on screening by digital examination of rectum. Definitive diagnosis is expensive (serum tumour markers, ultrasound, biopsy). Recent studies raise serious questions regarding the benefits of early detection and surgical intervention before symptoms develop (USPSTF, 1989; Brawer et al., 1992). In studies in the USA, men of African origin and men with a family history of prostate cancer appeared to be at greater risk; these groups should therefore be given priority for screening (USPSTF, 1989).

Resource levels required. Medium for detection by digital rectal examination, high for biopsy; high for surgery.

● Skin cancer

Screening for skin cancer in the general population is not recommended. In areas of high prevalence, education of the public in primary prevention (use of sunscreen products, hats and other protective clothing) and in early detection (self-referral for suspicious lesions) is more rational.

Resource levels required. Low for screening by inspection of exposed skin by primary care workers, but the technique needs validation; high for biopsy and surgery.

● Liver cancer

Screening is not recommended. No accurate screening test exists, and there is no evidence of any benefit from early detection. Emphasis should be on primary prevention through community-wide action for the prevention of hepatitis B infection, especially in infants (see page 68).

Summary tables

Key to terms and abbreviations used

The tables on the following pages summarize the recommendations discussed in the text and the key points leading to these recommendations. The following terms are used frequently in the summary tables. Other terms and abbreviations used both in the tables and text are defined in the Glossary, page 165.

Recommended. It is recommended that high priority be given to considering the use of screening of asymptomatic persons or persons with unrecognized health problems as part of a primary health care approach to prevention for the problem under consideration, in most cases as an adjunct to primary prevention.

Uncertain. Recommendation uncertain regarding use of screening of asymptomatic persons as part of a primary health care approach to prevention for the problem under consideration.

Not recommended. It is not recommended to give priority to the use of screening of asymptomatic persons as part of a primary health care approach to prevention for the problem under consideration.

Early detection recommended. The screening of asymptomatic persons may not be appropriate, but early detection of signs or symptoms is recommended as a priority in a primary health care approach to prevention for this problem, generally as an adjunct to primary prevention.

Low resource level. Can be done by enquiry or inspection without instruments or a laboratory, or with very simple instruments and materials; does not require professional or highly technical training.

Medium resource level. Requires basic instruments or laboratory facilities typically found at a health centre; requires nonspecialized technical or professional training.

High resource level. Requires technology generally available only at district or hospital level, or requires specialized technical or professional training.

Very high resource level. Requires technology or training generally not available at district level but only at national or regional referral centre.

Table 1. Screening in prenatal care

Health problem or risk factor	Recommendation on use of screening	Resource levels required			Comments
		Screening	Definitive diagnosis	Effective timely intervention	
Prior complication of pregnancy, labour or delivery; or prior adverse pregnancy outcome	Recommended	Low (enquiry or inspection of home-based records)	Medium or high (referral to care provider with more training)	Medium or high (referral to care provider with more training or to centre with capacity for operative delivery)	
Age or parity indicating high risk	Recommended	Low (enquiry or inspection of home-based records)		Medium or high (referral to care provider with more training)	Referral to centre with capacity for operative delivery may be necessary.
Short stature	Recommended	Low (inspection with or without simple measuring device)	Medium (pelvic examination) or high (X-ray pelvimetry)	Medium or high (obstetric provider with more training or capacity for operative delivery if obstructed labour)	Women at risk for obstructed labour should be near facility with operative capacity in last 1–2 months of pregnancy.
Maternal immunization status (tetanus; rubella)	Recommended	Low (enquiry or inspection of home-based records)	Medium (to measure rubella antibody titre)	Low (tetanus immunization; advice regarding need for post-partum rubella immunization)	
Psychosocial and socioeconomic risks in the household	Recommended (screening and early detection) Research priority: accurate methods for risk assessment at primary care level	Low or medium (enquiry and observation, especially in home but uncertain validity with unskilled observer)	Uncertain	Uncertain; may be low or medium (social support, supportive counselling, or social services for some problems)	Timely identification of risks with early intervention can improve maternal and child health outcome. Effective intervention may involve action at individual, family, or community level. Primary prevention should be the highest priority.

Barriers to access to health care services	Recommended (as an adjunct to primary prevention of access problems including outreach to populations with special barriers)	Low (enquiry)		Low (outreach; additional surveillance and support)	Early identification of geographical, financial, or other access problems should inform plans for follow-up with those who make an initial visit but are at risk of subsequent underutilization. Primary prevention is most important, including outreach to achieve universal coverage.
Smoking, use of alcohol, or other harmful substance by expectant mother	Early detection recommended as adjunct to primary prevention. Research priority: effective primary care intervention	Low (enquiry and review of records)		Low, medium, or high (social support or counselling services for mother; treatment for infants of drug-dependent mothers)	Primary prevention should be emphasized. Screening is a minor adjunct to public health measures including education, legislation, and accessible treatment services.
Poor maternal nutritional status, weight gain; poor fetal growth	Recommended only where adequate supplementation and effective counselling are available	Low (scales for weight gain; measuring-tape for fundal height)	Low or medium (laboratory tests) or high (ultrasound)	Low or medium (counselling, supplementation) or high (referral to high-risk centre if low birth weight anticipated)	Screening is a minor adjunct to multisectoral efforts to promote adequate food supply and intake. Doubtful effectiveness of counselling individuals when problem is community-wide. Not recommended: routine ultrasound for determination of gestational age.
Occupational risks, e.g., woman performs heavy labour, or is exposed to teratogens	Uncertain	Low (enquiry)	Variable	Variable	Primary prevention should be emphasized. Counselling individuals on risks may not be effective without action at policy level to remove hazards and exposures. Community involvement (e.g., through labour unions) essential.

Table 1. Screening in prenatal care (continued)

Health problem or risk factor	Recommendation on use of screening	Resource levels required			Comments
		Screening	Definitive diagnosis	Effective timely intervention	
History of chronic disease or recent neglected symptoms suggesting acute illness requiring treatment	Early detection recommended	Low (enquiry; record review) or medium	Medium or high, depending on condition	Low, medium, or high, depending on condition	Screening and individual treatment should not be a substitute for primary prevention at community level.
Iron deficiency anaemia	Recommended	Low or medium (haemoglobin/ haematocrit)	Low (positive response to iron) or medium	Low (iron or dietary supplement)	Primary prevention most important. Early detection of persons with symptoms also recommended.
Malaria	Recommended in areas where malaria is endemic as adjunct to primary prevention	Low or medium (blood smear)	Low or medium	Low or medium (chloroquine or other medication)	
Iodine deficiency	Not recommended	High (blood or urine assays)	High (blood or urine assays)	Low (iodine supplement)	Universal iodine supplementation is recommended in communities with high prevalence of iodine deficiency. Screening and treating asymptomatic individuals relatively inefficient in such settings. Periodic monitoring should be done at population level to identify communities that need supplementation. Early detection of thyroid enlargement by physical examination should be part of antenatal care. See Congenital hypothyroidism in Table 2.

Multiple gestation, breech or transverse lie	Recommended	Low (abdominal examination) or medium (pelvic examination by skilled examiner)	Medium (more skilled examiner) or high (ultrasound examination)	Medium or high (suspicion requires referral to district/hospital level for possible operative delivery)	Important treatable cause of maternal and fetal morbidity and mortality.
Hypertensive disease of pregnancy	Recommended	Low (blood pressure cuff and stethoscope; dipstick for urine)	Low	Low, medium, or high	Important risk factor for premature labour. Primary prevention by education of girls and women on perineal hygiene.
Asymptomatic bacteriuria	Recommended	Low or medium (urinalysis or urine culture; dipsticks can identify leukocytes without microscopic examination)	Medium in most cases (unless need for diagnosis of repeated infections or failure to respond to treatment)	Low or medium, in most cases	
Asymptomatic gonorrhoea or chlamydial infection	Recommended	Low (urine dipstick for pyuria) or medium (urinalysis for leukocytes, or abnormal vaginal/cervical discharge or cervical erosion on examination)	Medium or high (culture). May be reasonable to treat presumptively on screening results if definitive diagnosis not feasible.	Low or medium (oral antibiotics)	Primary prevention through education on safe sex most important.
Syphilis	Recommended	Medium or high technology but low cost (VDRL test)	Medium or high technology but low cost (RPR test)	Medium (antibiotics)	Testing and treatment are relatively inexpensive compared with costs and consequences of disease. Primary prevention through education on safe sex most important.

Table 1. Screening in prenatal care (*continued*)

Health problem or risk factor	Recommendation on use of screening	Resource levels required		Effective timely intervention	Comments
		Screening	Definitive diagnosis		
HIV infection or disease	Uncertain (see p. 67). Recommended only when voluntary, when skilled pre- and post-test counselling is provided, and when therapeutic abortion would be a likely option for those with infection	Medium or high, including skilled pre-test counselling	Medium or high	Low to very high, including skilled post-test counselling and option of therapeutic abortion, and treatment for substance abusers	Highest priority needs to be primary prevention through promotion of safe sex.
Hepatitis B infection	Recommended for communities with vertical transmission and HBsAg prevalence < 10%	Medium (testing for surface antigen)	Medium or high (including tests for infectivity)	Medium or high (hepatitis B immune globulin to infant of infected mother; costs may be low if vaccine provided by public sector)	If prevalence in community is ≥ 10%, it may be more rational to immunize universally without individual screening. Primary prevention through promotion of safe sex and preventing transmission through contaminated needles is also important.
ABO blood group	Recommended, giving first priority to those at highest risk for transfusion, if unable to screen all	Medium or high		High (transfusion)	Prioritize those at risk for operative delivery or haemorrhage.
Rhesus (Rh) antibodies	Recommended but prioritize conditions listed above	Medium or high		High (Rh immune globulin to Rh − mother of Rh + fetus)	Recommended but may not be affordable at present.

Gestational diabetes	Not recommended for general population of pregnant women; screen high-risk subgroups	Medium	Medium or high (requires multiple postprandial blood glucose measurements)	Low or medium	Accurate testing expensive. Targeted screening of obese women and those with prior macrosomic baby should be a priority.
Electronic fetal monitoring for fetal asphyxia	Not recommended	High	High	High	Great expense; uncertain benefits; substantial increase in operative delivery associated with use.
Prenatal genetic screening					Highly specialized resources needed for counselling and follow-up as well as testing.
(a) Chromosomal abnormalities or direct evidence of structural abnormalities	Not recommended	High or very high, including skilled pre-test counselling	Very high (referral hospital only; ultrasound not sufficiently sensitive)	Medium (therapeutic abortion), high or very high (referral hospital), including skilled post-test counselling	Safety and efficacy of routine ultrasound in pregnancy not established. Primary prevention should be emphasized, e.g., discouraging births to women over 35 years and avoiding toxic exposure.
(b) Haemoglobinopathies and other inherited diseases detectable by prenatal biochemical assays	Not recommended (see Table 3). Targeted screening of high-risk subgroups may be worth while where the health services are adequately developed.	Medium for sickle-cell testing, high for other conditions. Skilled pre-test counselling may require high resource level	High or very high	High or very high (and yield uncertain)	Total expense of effective strategy will be out of reach in places with limited resources. See Table 3, Sickle-cell disease.

Table 2. Screening in reproductive/family health care

Health problem or risk factor	Recommendation on use of screening	Resource levels required			Comments
		Screening	Definitive diagnosis	Effective timely intervention	
Risk of unintended or high-risk pregnancy in future	Recommended as part of routine pre-natal and postpartum care. "Opportunistic" screening should also be integrated into all other routine care for children (targeting parents), young people, and adults.	Low (enquiry or in-spection of reproduc-tive history in home-based mother's record)		Low, medium, or high	Screening is a minor adjunct to public education and provision of safe, acceptable, and accessible family planning methods.
STDs including HIV infection	Opportunistic screen-ing, case-finding, and early detection recommended for those at high risk, according to local epidemiology, as an adjunct to promotion of safe sex	Medium, including pre-test counselling for HIV testing	Medium or high	Low (counselling to prevent further spread of STDs), medium or high, including post-test counselling for HIV-positive persons	Screening is an adjunct to pub-lic education and promotion of safe sex and provision of accessible and acceptable services for diagnosis and treatment.

Cervical cancer (see also Table 7, p. 163)

(a) High-risk groups (≥ 35 years, STDs, or high parity)	(a) Recommended to screen with cytology	(a) High (cervical cytology: taking specimen requires medium resources only but reading smear requires highly skilled cytotechnician) and well developed communication system	(a) High (biopsy)	(a) High (cone biopsy or more extensive surgery) or very high if extensive invasion (radiation therapy)	(a) and (b) Trained cytotechnicians are often scarce even at district hospital or national level. Where treatment capabilities for advanced cases are limited, at least palliation and pain control should be guaranteed. Current practice of frequent screening of low-risk women < 35 years is not rational. Ensure coverage of high-risk groups, including women over 35 (currently widely neglected), before screening low-risk groups. Primary prevention: education on safe sex; family planning; prevent tobacco use.
(b) Others	(b) Uncertain; recommended but as lower priority and with less frequency than among high risk groups. Research priority validation of accurate low-cost methods of screening	(b) Low or medium (visual inspection of cervix — not yet fully validated but appears promising)	(b) High (biopsy)	(b) High (cone biopsy or more extensive surgery) or very high if extensive invasion (radiation therapy)	
Reproductive hazards in workplace or home	Uncertain	Low (enquiry or observation) but requires trained personnel; medium or high if tests required	Low, medium, or high	Uncertain; removal of hazard may require change in policy	Primary prevention with protective regulations and routine surveillance of workplaces and of commercial and residential areas should be the highest priority.

Table 3. Screening in health care of newborns

Health problem or risk factor	Recommendation on use of screening	Resource levels required			Comments
		Screening	Definitive diagnosis	Effective timely intervention	
Low birth weight	Early detection recommended	Low	Low (scales)	Low, medium, or high	Excellent marker for generally at-risk infant/young child. Primary prevention essential through general community-wide health promotion and through family planning and comprehensive prenatal care.
Maternal/household psychosocial and socio-economic risks	Screening and early detection recommended Research priority: low-cost primary care methods of early detection and intervention	Low (observation and transfer of information from mother's to infant's records)	Low or medium	Low, medium, or high, depending on problem (counselling, support, and referral to appropriate services)	Adjunct to primary prevention through family planning, comprehensive prenatal care, and general socioeconomic development of community
Congenital syphilis	Uncertain recommendation on screening newborns; prenatal screening recommended	Medium	Medium	Low or medium (parenteral antibiotics)	Prevention through prenatal screening and treatment is a higher priority. Newborns in high-risk subgroups should be screened even if prenatal test negative.
Undescended testis	Uncertain for newborn (recommended by age one year)	Medium (low technology, but skilled examiner)	Medium	High (surgery)	Screening and intervention recommended at age one year unless prior examination normal

Condition	Recommendation	Technology		Resources	Comments
Congenital hypothyroidism	Uncertain	Medium (test of cord blood on filter-paper sent to central laboratory)	Medium or high	Low (iodine supplementation)	Primary prevention essential. Universal supplementation with iodine should be provided in communities with high prevalence and should be higher priority than screening.
Congenital dislocation of hip	Uncertain recommendation on screening newborn; recommended in early toddler stage	Medium (low technology but highly skilled examiner)	Medium or high	High (orthopaedic referral and possibly surgery)	Detection easier and intervention effective around age two years.
Treatable abnormalities of head circumference	Not recommended unless definitive diagnosis and treatment available for all with positive screen	Low to medium (doubtful reliability without highly skilled examiner)	High or very high	High or very high (referral hospital with neurosurgical capability)	Relatively rare. Definitive diagnosis and treatment very expensive. Not recommended if definitive diagnosis and treatment cannot be provided for all with positive screen, or if more common conditions have not yet been addressed.
Asymptomatic cardiac abnormality	Uncertain	Medium (low technology but highly skilled examiner)	High or very high	Medium technology but expensive because long-term (antibiotic prophylaxis), or very high (cardiac surgery)	Long-term antibiotic prophylaxis is expensive, as is surgery. Many abnormalities will produce symptoms and lead to early detection. Primary prevention of anomalies should be a higher priority.
Haemoglobinopathies: (a) Sickle cell	Uncertain	Medium (sickling test is simple but requires laboratory and pre-test counselling)		High (intensive hospital care for infections in homozygote); genetic counselling for heterozygote	Early identification of sickle-cell disease may save life through more appropriate early treatment, but treatment is expensive and intensive. No evidence that identification in newborn leads to changes in reproductive decisions.

Table 3. Screening in health care of newborns (*continued*)

Health problem or risk factor	Recommendation on use of screening	Resource levels required		Effective timely intervention	Comments
		Screening	Definitive diagnosis		
(b) Other haemo-globinopathies	Not recommended	High	High	No effective early intervention for homozygotes; only intervention for heterozygotes is genetic counselling	No evidence for effectiveness of genetic counselling after testing of newborn.
Phenylketonuria	Uncertain; not recommended as a high priority where resources are very constrained	High	High	Medium but dietary counselling of uncertain effectiveness where access to special foods is limited	Rare condition. Testing is expensive and logistically difficult. Intervention of uncertain effectiveness.
Other inborn errors of metabolism	Not recommended	High	High or very high	Variable, but generally high or very high	Very rare. Low yield from screening of newborns.
Eye abnormalities not observable without special instruments	Uncertain	Medium (red reflex with ophthalmoscope)	High	High or very high	Primary prevention of congenital anomalies is preferable. Conditions for which early detection would allow effective intervention are rare.

Table 4. Screening in care of infants and children under 6 years of age (see also Table 6)

Health problem or risk factor	Recommendation on use of screening	Resource levels required			Comments
		Screening	Definitive diagnosis	Effective timely intervention	
At-risk infant or preschool child	Screening and early detection recommended Research priorities: development and validation of primary care methods of detection and intervention	Low (by enquiry or inspection of records; history of low birth weight an excellent marker; inadequate immunization status may also be a good marker)	Low, medium or high for complete assessment of complex problem	Low, medium, or high, depending on problem	Primary prevention essential. Assessment of risks and plan for intervention may require special training and referral resources. Community-based approaches to detection of, and intervention with, common risks should be a high priority for research. Screening and intervention with household-level risks is only an adjunct to community-wide and household-level prevention through multisectoral actions.
Immunization status	Recommended	Low (enquiry or inspection of home-based child's record)		Low or medium (immunization)	Inadequate immunization status may be a marker for the generally at-risk child.
Monitoring of physical growth	Uncertain recommendation on screening low-risk children; detection of the generally at-risk child (see above) should be priority	Low	Medium, high, or very high	Low, medium, high, or very high	Emphasis should be on primary prevention of malnutrition and early detection of children suspected to have problems. Uncertain yield from monitoring individuals where problem is community-wide or resources are inadequate to intervene effectively even with individuals.

Table 4. Screening in care of infants and children under 6 years of age (*continued*)

Health problem or risk factor	Recommendation on use of screening	Resource levels required			Comments
		Screening	Definitive diagnosis	Effective timely intervention	
Mental, neurological, or psychosocial development	Recommended at primary care level; formal developmental testing not recommended	Low (developmental milestones checked by primary care worker)	Medium, high, or very high	Medium, high, or very high	Primary prevention should be emphasized. Intervention may require specialist, generally at district hospital or higher referral level. Primary care interventions may minimize handicaps and prevent child abuse.
Congenital dislocation of hip	Recommended in toddlers	Low (observe gait)	Medium or high	High (specialist, possibly surgery)	Assessment in infant difficult before walking: easier in toddler.
Visual problems	Screening for squint and amblyopia recommended by age 3. Screening for visual acuity not recommended before school entry	Low or medium (observation; enquiry of parents, but skilled and trained examiner required)	Medium or high	Medium, high, or very high	Early intervention for strabismus or amblyopia essential to prevent blindness.
Hearing problems	Screening not recommended; early detection recommended	No accurate low-cost screening test	Medium or high	Low to medium (treat otitis); high or very high (surgery or hearing aid); alternative: supportive measures to minimize handicap (low)	Accurate low-cost screening test lacking. Definitive treatment expensive. Yield uncertain. Early detection of problems by parents and child care workers recommended.
Undescended testis	Recommended	Low or medium technology but requires training	Medium (skilled examiner)	High (surgery)	Intervention around one year of age to reduce infertility; surgery may or may not reduce risk of testicular cancer.

Condition					
Treatable abnormalities of head circumference in infant	Uncertain	Low or medium (but doubtful accuracy of screening measurements)	High	High or very high	Relatively rare conditions. Definitive diagnosis and intervention very expensive. Not recommended if definitive diagnosis and treatment cannot be provided for all with positive screen, or if more common conditions have not yet been addressed.
Asymptomatic bacteriuria	Not recommended	Low or medium (dipstick or urinalysis)	Medium or high (culture)	Medium or high (but uncertain impact on health)	High expense of testing with uncertain yield.
Subclinical iron deficiency anaemia and lead poisoning	Not recommended	Medium	Medium or high	Low (diet change or iron supplement) or low, medium, or high (removal of lead exposure)	Clinical significance uncertain. Emphasize primary prevention through community-wide promotion of good nutrition and removal of environmental lead.
Rheumatic heart disease and other asymptomatic cardiac abnormalities	Not recommended as a priority	Medium (but many false positives)	High or very high	Medium (long-term antibiotic prophylaxis is expensive), high, or very high (cardiac surgery)	Many false positives on screening with danger of false labelling. Primary prevention through early detection and treatment of streptococcal infection and prevention of birth defects.
Elevated blood cholesterol	Not recommended	Medium	Medium or high (multiple measurements needed)	Low, medium, or high (yield uncertain)	Need for multiple determinations to establish definitive diagnosis. Primary prevention of coronary artery disease should be emphasized.
High blood pressure	Not recommended	Low	Low or medium (for laboratory work-up to determine etiology)	Medium (but expensive long-term)	Very rare in young children. Emphasize primary prevention of cardiovascular and cerebrovascular disease.

Table 5. Screening in care of school-age children and adolescents (see also Table 6)

Health problem or risk factor	Recommendation on use of screening	Resource levels required			Comments
		Screening	Definitive diagnosis	Effective timely intervention	
Problems of growth and development	Recommended on school entry; early detection of problems recommended thereafter, without formal screening	Low (assessment by teachers according to local norms)	Medium or high	Low, medium, high, or very high, depending on the problem	Teachers should be trained to recognize developmental, learning, and psychosocial problems and refer appropriately. Primary prevention should be emphasized.
	Research priority: low-cost primary care methods of early detection and intervention				
Immunization status	Recommended on school entry and later according to local schedules	Low (enquiry or inspection of home-based card)		Low (vaccination)	Immunizations are low-cost and of proven effectiveness. Inadequate immunization status may be good marker for the generally high-risk child.
Visual problems	Recommended on school entry; uncertain recommendation on frequency of repeat screening	Low (can be done by teachers)	Medium (definitive diagnosis of refractive errors)	Low (simple precautions to minimize learning problems) or medium (glasses)	Early detection of learning problems also important.
Hearing problems	Not recommended; early detection of problems recommended	Low for early detection (observation by teachers or parents); medium or high for formal screening	High or very high	Low for simple tactics such as favourable seating in classroom. Medium, high, or very high.	Accurate formal screening test is not available for mass testing. Early detection of problems by teachers and parents is recommended.

Oral health problems	Not recommended	Low	Medium	Medium	Emphasis should be on primary prevention through education on hygiene and through fluoridation.
Sexually transmitted diseases (including HIV infection) in sexually active adolescents	Recommended annually or with frequency according to likely exposures	Medium (but may involve central laboratory)	Medium or high	Low or medium	Confidentiality in testing and treatment is essential. Primary prevention through education on safe sex is essential.
Risk of pregnancy in school-age children	"Opportunistic" screening recommended for all adolescents	Low (enquiry)		Low or medium (education, contraception)	All pregnancies in adolescents are high-risk for mother and child. All adolescents should be asked whether they are sexually active and, if so, whether they use any method of protection. Regardless of reply, they should also be asked if they have any questions about sex, birth control, or sexually transmitted diseases. Screening is an adjunct to primary prevention through public education on safe sex and family planning and general socioeconomic development.
Subclinical iron deficiency anaemia	Not recommended for general population; recommended for pregnant women of any age	Low or medium (haemoglobin or haematocrit)	Low (response to iron) or medium (serum iron studies)	Low (uncertain clinical significance of mild iron deficiency in children or non-pregnant adolescents)	For pregnant adolescents only (see Table 1).

Table 5. Screening in care of school-age children and adolescents (*continued*)

Health problem or risk factor	Recommendation on use of screening	Resource levels required			Comments
		Screening	Definitive diagnosis	Effective timely intervention	
Scoliosis	Not recommended	Low, accuracy doubtful (physical examination unreliable; many false positives)	High	High (doubtful effectiveness except in extreme cases that are likely to be symptomatic)	Screening tests inaccurate. Treatability and significance of subtle scoliosis doubtful. Marked cases should be noted by observation without special manoeuvre. Early detection recommended.
High blood pressure	Not recommended in this age group	Low	Low or medium (laboratory tests and examination to determine etiology)	Medium technology, but very expensive long-term	Emphasis should be on primary prevention of high blood pressure and cardiovascular disease.
Elevated blood cholesterol	Not recommended	Medium	Medium or high	Low, medium, or high; effectiveness doubtful	Emphasis should be on primary prevention of coronary heart disease.
Tuberculosis	Not recommended for asymptomatic persons where BCG prophylaxis makes tuberculin testing unhelpful	Low (enquiry regarding symptoms or history of exposure) or medium	Medium (sputum) or high (X-ray)	Medium	Routine X-rays of asymptomatic persons not recommended. Emphasis should be on public education and early detection of symptomatic or exposed persons, along with primary prevention. If BCG not given, tuberculin screening can be a useful adjunct.
Asymptomatic bacteriuria	Not recommended except among pregnant adolescents	Low or medium (urinalysis or urine culture)	Medium (culture) or high (radiographic studies of urinary tract)	Low or medium (antibiotics) but uncertain impact on health outcome except in pregnancy	Pyuria may be a screen for STD in males.

156

Schistosomiasis of urinary tract	Uncertain	Low (enquiry regarding symptoms, gross inspection for haematuria, or reagent strips)	Medium	Low or medium	Treatment ineffective without environmental measures to prevent reinfection. Primary prevention should be the highest priority.
Cancer (a) Testicular	Not recommended for general population	Low (self-examination) or medium	High	High (surgery and chemotherapy)	Emphasis should be on education of public to practise self-referral. Screen those with history of undescended testis even if surgically repaired.
(b) Cervical	Not recommended as a high priority for general population in this age group	Low or medium (inspection of cervix) or high (cytology)	High	High or very high	Screening those with STDs a high priority. Cervical cancer is extremely rare in adolescents. See Table 7 and pp. 131–134.
Haemoglobinopathies (including sickle cell trait)	Not recommended	High, including pre- and post-test counselling (although sickling test itself is simple)	High or very high	Homozygote would be detected earlier. No evidence for effectiveness of genetic counselling of heterozygotes as part of routine services.	No evidence that screening leads to changes in reproductive decisions. See recommendations on screening newborns for sickle-cell disease (Table 3).
Rheumatic heart disease	Not recommended	Medium (many false positives)	High	Medium (but expensive), high, or very high (cardiac surgery)	Screening requires highly skilled examiner; definitive diagnosis and long-term antibiotic prophylaxis expensive.

Table 6. Screening of children and adults for communicable diseases

Health problem or risk factor	Recommendation on use of screening	Resource levels required			Comments
		Screening	Definitive diagnosis	Effective timely intervention	
Sexually transmitted diseases	Recommended for high-risk groups and pregnant women; early detection of risks, exposure, or symptoms recommended	Low (enquiry regarding risks or symptoms) or medium to high (laboratory testing)	Medium or high	Low or medium (antibiotics)	Confidentiality in testing and follow-up is essential. Screening is an adjunct to public education regarding safe sexual practices and provision of accessible and acceptable services.
HIV infection	Uncertain	Medium or high, including pretest counselling	Medium or high	Medium or high, including skilled post-test counselling. Supportive social services may be provided at a primary care level and can have a major impact on quality of life for an HIV-infected individual.	Highest priority needs to be primary prevention through promotion of safe sexual practices, use of clean needles and prevention of drug abuse.
Malaria	Not recommended for asymptomatic persons (except pregnant women in endemic areas); early detection of symptoms recommended	Low or medium (blood smears)	Medium	Low or medium (chloroquine/other medication)	Primary prevention is essential. Public education to promote self-referral for symptoms (early detection) may be more productive than mass screening.

Disease				
Tuberculosis	Not recommended for asymptomatic persons where BCG vaccination is the norm; early detection of symptoms recommended	Medium (sputum smears; tuberculin testing not helpful with BCG history) or high (X-ray)	Medium or high	Medium (medication)	Mass screening has generally low yield in absence of suggestive symptoms or history. Emphasis should be on primary prevention along with early detection of persons with symptoms and treatment of household contacts of cases.
Leprosy, leishmaniasis, filariasis, and other endemic diseases with skin manifestations	Not recommended; early detection of symptoms recommended	Low (inspection for typical lesions)	Medium or high	Medium or high	Public education to promote self-referral for characteristic skin lesions is more productive than mass screening. Self-referral depends on public education and accessible and acceptable medical services.
Schistosomiasis	Not recommended; early detection of symptoms recommended	Low (enquiry, gross inspection of urine, or testing urine with reagent strip for blood)	Medium	Medium (medication) but effectiveness doubtful without prevention of reinfection	Emphasis should be on primary prevention and self-referral for symptoms. See Table 5. Monitoring and intervention should occur at community level.
Onchocerciasis and trachoma	Not recommended; early detection of symptoms recommended	Low (inspection for typical lesion)	High	High	Vector control (primary prevention) most important for onchocerciasis; hygiene important for trachoma. Self-referral for symptoms (early detection) also important for both of these major causes of preventable blindness.

Table 7. Screening in health care of adults (see also Table 6)

Health problem or risk factor	Recommendation on use of screening	Resource levels required			Comments
		Screening	Definitive diagnosis	Effective timely intervention	
General health problems					
Dental or periodontal disease	Recommended	Low	Medium	Medium	Common cause of significant suffering and disability in adults. Primary prevention through public education on hygiene is essential with special emphasis on educating children.
Risk of unintended or high-risk pregnancy (see also Table 2)	"Opportunistic" screening and early detection recommended	Low (enquiry or inspection of reproductive history on home-based card)		Low or medium, generally; high if surgical contraception desired	Screening is a minor adjunct to public education and provision of safe, acceptable, and accessible family planning services.
Psychosocial problems including domestic violence and alcohol and drug abuse	Uncertain ("opportunistic" screening); early detection of household risks for children recommended Research priority: low-cost primary care assessment methods and interventions	Low (observation or enquiry)	Low or medium	Low, medium, or high	Screening is a minor adjunct to other preventive measures. Assessment requires training. Intervention may require referral resources, but simple interventions to mobilize additional social support may be effective. Primary prevention should be emphasized.

Problem	Recommendation				Comments
Problems of functional status in the elderly	Recommended. Research priority: low-cost primary care assessment methods and interventions	Low (observation, especially in home)	Low or medium	Low or medium	Functional status may often be improved by simple interventions, including mobilizing additional social support and arranging household items to aid mobility and decrease hazards.
Cataracts and refractive errors	Screening recommended in elderly; early detection of problems recommended for other adults	Low (enquiry or simple assessment of acuity)	Medium (optometric evaluation)	High (cataract extraction or corrective lenses)	Cataracts are a leading cause of reversible blindness in elderly who often consider limited vision normal with aging.
Glaucoma	Not recommended as a priority for general population	Medium or high	High	Medium or high	No accurate primary care screening test. Value of early intervention in most asymptomatic persons questionable. (Screen high-risk groups.)
Occupational hazards	Uncertain	Low (enquiry)	Medium or high (laboratory tests)	Uncertain, removal of hazard may require action at policy level	Primary prevention by monitoring workplaces should be emphasized. Screening may be a useful adjunct, but of secondary importance

Cardiovascular and cerebrovascular disease

USPSTF recommended against routine mass screening with ECG, chest X-ray, blood lipid profiles, and auscultation for carotid bruits.

Problem	Recommendation				Comments
Risks associated with diet, exercise, or substance use, including tobacco	Not recommended. Research priority: effective preventive measures	Low (enquiry)		Low or medium (counselling)	Emphasis should be on primary prevention and making treatment available. Approach must be country-specific.

Table 7. Screening in health care of adults (*continued*)

Health problem or risk factor	Recommendation on use of screening	Resource levels required			Comments
		Screening	Definitive diagnosis	Effective timely intervention	
High blood pressure	Uncertain; not recommended in general population when resources for treatment are inadequate. Targeted screening of highest-risk groups recommended when resources for intervention assured Research priority: primary prevention and low-cost acceptable treatment	Low	Low or medium (laboratory and examination)	Medium technology but costly over long-term	Screening is relatively simple, but long-term treatment is expensive with compliance problems. Thresholds for treatment with medication may need to be higher in areas of high prevalence with limited resources. Broad public health efforts to reduce risk (tobacco, diet, exercise) are essential and should be top priority.
Elevated blood cholesterol	Not recommended in general population	Medium	Medium (repeated measurements required; expensive)	Low or medium (diet counselling) or medium (medication is expensive); yield of treatment uncertain in most populations	If resources are available for definitive diagnosis and intervention, it is rational to prioritize screening for those with family history of early coronary artery disease.
Carotid bruits	Not recommended in asymptomatic persons	Medium or high (auscultation by trained listener)	Very high (arteriogram)	Very high (carotid endarterectomy)	Definitive diagnosis and treatment extremely expensive. Uncertain benefit of early intervention in asymptomatic persons. Emphasis should be on primary prevention.

Elevated blood sugar (diabetes mellitus; glucose intolerance)	Not recommended in asymptomatic persons	Medium	Medium	Medium; not clear that intervention in asymptomatic non-pregnant adults would improve outcome	Mass screening of asymptomatic adults is not rational.
Cancer					
Cervical cancer (a) High-risk groups (≥ 35 years, STDs, or high parity)	Recommended to screen with cytology	High (cervical cytology: taking specimen requires only medium resources but reading smear requires highly skilled cytotechnician and well-developed communication system)	High	Low or medium for pain control. High (cone biopsy or more extensive surgery) or very high if extensive invasion (radiation therapy)	Trained cytotechnicians are often scarce even at district hospital or national level. Where treatment capabilities for advanced cases are limited, palliation and pain control at least should be guaranteed. Current practice of frequent screening of low-risk women < 35 years is not rational. Ensure coverage of high-risk groups, including women over 35 (currently widely neglected), before screening low-risk groups. Primary prevention: education on safe sex; family planning; prevention of tobacco use.
(b) Others	Recommended but as lower priority and with less frequency than among high-risk groups

Research priority: validation of accurate low-cost methods of screening | Low or medium (visual inspection of cervix not yet fully validated but appears promising) | | | |
| Breast cancer in women | Uncertain recommendation on screening; early detection recommended

Research priority: accurate low-cost methods of screening and early detection | Low (self-examination), medium (clinical examination), or high (mammography) | High (mammography or biopsy) | High (surgery with or without chemotherapy); very high for radiation therapy | Public education to promote self-examination appears important to achieve earlier self-referral. Mammography excellent over age of 50, but probably too expensive for population screening in most developing countries. |

Table 7. Screening in health care of adults (*continued*)

Health problem or risk factor	Recommendation on use of screening	Resource levels required			Comments
		Screening	Definitive diagnosis	Effective timely intervention	
Oral cancer	Recommended in high prevalence areas	Low (can be done by primary care workers)	Medium or high	Medium or high	Community-based approaches successful.
Colorectal cancer	Not recommended as a priority	Medium (faecal occult blood or digital rectal examination) or high (sigmoidoscopy)	High (X-ray and biopsy)	High (surgery)	Screening by low-cost methods is extremely inaccurate. Sigmoidoscopy is relatively expensive and of low acceptability to the public. Primary prevention through high-fibre diet.
Prostate cancer	Not recommended as a priority	Medium (digital rectal examination)	High (biopsy)	High (surgery)	Benefits of early intervention for asymptomatic prostatic cancers uncertain.
Skin cancer	Not recommended	Low (inspection of exposed skin)	High (biopsy)	High (surgery)	Emphasis should be on primary prevention and self-referral for suspicious lesions.
Liver cancer	Not recommended				No test available for screening adults. See Table 1, Hepatitis B infection.

Glossary of terms used in this publication[1]

Case-finding. The detection of adverse health conditions or disease (symptomatic or not) in people who present for services for other reasons. Case-finding has sometimes been called "opportunistic" screening because it takes advantage of an opportunity created by circumstances. While there can be some overlap between case-finding and screening, this publication generally distinguishes between case-finding, which is clinically based (i.e., offered to users of clinical services) and often identifies persons with symptomatic disease, and screening, which should be population-based and seeks out asymptomatic persons, ideally before disease has occurred.

Community-based. Located in the community where the target population for services lives or works.

Community-oriented. Addressing the needs of a specific community and involving active participation by members of that community. Sometimes used (imprecisely) interchangeably with community-based.

Detection. The identification of health risks or disease. A broad term encompassing screening, diagnosis, and early detection.

> **• Early detection.** A general term encompassing case-finding, health screening, and other approaches to the identification of a health risk or disease sufficiently early in its course to prevent or minimize damage. Any early detection procedure can be thought of as a test; it does not necessarily involve the use of laboratory procedures. It may or may not be diagnostic.

District health system. A more or less self-contained segment of a national health system taking responsibility for the health care of a well defined population living within a clearly delineated geographical and administrative area. A district's population is usually between 50 000 and 500 000 persons. Usually, a district health system has a general hospital with inpatient and outpatient services providing support at the referral level for the health care facilities (health centres and peripheral health posts) within the district.

---

[1] The definitions given here apply to the use of terms in this publication, and are not necessarily applicable in other contexts.

Family health care. *See* Reproductive health care.

Health for all. A phrase summing up the goal adopted at the Thirty-first World Health Assembly in 1978: the attainment by all the people of the world by the year 2000 of a level of health that will permit them to lead a socially and economically productive life.

Health promotion. Fostering of lifestyles and other social, economic, environmental and personal factors conducive to health.

Health screening. Use of presumptive methods to detect unrecognized health risks or asymptomatic disease in order to permit timely intervention. Health screening is a particular kind of early detection practice, in which inapparent risk factors or unrecognized disease are actively looked for . A screening procedure can be thought of as a test; it does not necessarily involve the use of laboratory procedures. Screening procedures are generally easier to perform and cheaper than diagnostic procedures; their results are usually presumptive, and require confirmation through definitive diagnostic tests. While the term "health screening" is sometimes used more broadly, this publication deals with prescriptive screening, i.e., screening carried out with the purpose of targeting timely interventions at those found to have conditions requiring care.

• **Targeted screening.** Screening of selected subpopulations according to prior knowledge of which groups are at greatest risk (e.g., screening for cervical cancer of women who are over 35 years of age, have a history of sexually transmitted diseases, or have high parity). Targeted screening will have the greatest predictive value, because it is directed at relatively high-prevalence populations.

• **Untargeted (mass) screening.** Screening of whole population groups (generally defined by geographical criteria and perhaps broad age group or sex), without regard for whether the entire group is at significant risk for the condition (e.g., screening of all children for anaemia, all women of reproductive age for cervical cancer, or all adults for elevated blood lipid levels).

Health transition. The shift in the age distribution of the population that has occurred relatively recently in most developing countries, resulting in a higher proportion of elderly persons, accompanied by an increasing burden of chronic and noncommunicable disease.

Population-based. Addressing the needs of a defined population (often defined geographically, or by workplace, and at times by sex or broad age categories, but not by individuals' personal resources or history of using a particular health care facility). Population-based medical or health care addresses population-wide needs rather than only the needs of current users of services. One of the essential features of a primary health care approach is that it is population-based.

Predictive value. The predictive value of a detection procedure ("test") is its ability to distinguish persons with and without a condition. The predictive value is a function of the sensitivity and specificity (see below) of the test and the prevalence of the condition or risk factor in the population to be screened. A test that has high predictive values in one population may have lower predictive values in another; locally appropriate techniques for testing are needed as are locally appropriate standards for positive and negative results.

- **Negative predictive value** is the predictive value of a negative test. This is the likelihood that a negative test result is correct, i.e., that a person identified as not having a condition truly does not.

- **Positive predictive value** is the predictive value of a positive test. This is the likelihood that a positive test result is correct, i.e., that the person identified as having a condition truly has the condition. Even a relatively sensitive and specific test can have low positive predictive value if used in a population with a low prevalence of the condition being tested for.

Prevention. Measures to prevent adverse effects on health.

- **Primary prevention.** Prevention of disease or other health problems by intervening with causes and risk factors to prevent exposure, e.g., preventing infant diarrhoea by ensuring safe water supply and promoting breast-feeding; preventing cervical cancer by promoting safe sexual practices.

- **Secondary prevention.** Early detection and treatment of disease or precursors of disease, in order to limit its duration, severity, and sequelae, e.g., giving oral rehydration solution to an infant with diarrhoeal disease to promote recovery and prevent serious morbidity or mortality; detecting cervical dysplasia or carcinoma in situ to prevent invasive cervical carcinoma; controlling high blood pressure to prevent cardiovascular complications.

- **Tertiary prevention.** Measures to reduce the suffering, damage, or disability caused by established disease, e.g., teaching a victim of a cerebrovascular accident to recover speech and other functions lost; providing palliative care to reduce the pain or disability of a woman with disseminated invasive carcinoma of the cervix.

Primary care. Also called primary medical care. First-contact medical care services delivered by non-specialized personnel, generally in an outpatient setting. Commonly confused with primary health care (see below). *See also* Secondary care *and* Tertiary care.

Primary health care. Essential health care made accessible at a cost the country and community can afford, with methods that are practical, scientifically sound and socially acceptable. It is based on the following principles: equity; universal access to basic services, including primary and secondary medical care services; recognition of the multisectoral nature of health and disease determinants; community participation; and the promotion of health and well-being as opposed to the prevention or control of disease only.

Primary prevention. *See* Prevention.

Reproductive health care. Services to improve reproductive outcome and the health of people's reproductive organ systems. Includes family planning services. Sometimes called family health care.

Risk factor. A predisposing factor or precursor of disease or adverse health outcome.

Screening. *See* Health screening.

Secondary care. Secondary medical care. Care provided at the second level of contact in a health care system, ideally by referral from the primary care level. It is usually delivered in a hospital setting or by a specialist (e.g., general surgeon, obstetrician/gynaecologist, ophthalmologist).

Secondary prevention. *See* Prevention.

Sensitivity. The ability of a detection procedure to identify individuals having, or at risk of, conditions being sought; the proportion of true positives detected to be positive. A sensitive test has a low rate of false negative results but may have low positive predictive value if applied in a population with a low prevalence of the condition being tested for.

Specificity. The ability of a detection procedure to identify individuals not having and not at risk of conditions being sought; the proportion of true negatives identified as negative. A test that has high specificity has a low rate of false positives.

Tertiary care. Specialized medical care requiring services of a subspecialist and often a high degree of technology; may not be available at district level, but may require referral to resources at national or regional level.

Tertiary prevention. *See* Prevention.

Test. Any procedure (e.g., enquiry, physical examination, examination of individual health records, or laboratory procedure) used to detect health risks or disease.

References

Abeyewickreme I (1989) Cervical cytology screening in a sexually transmitted diseases clinic for the first time in Sri Lanka. *Genitourinary medicine*, 65: 98–102.

Al-Shawaf T et al. (1988) Gestational diabetes and impaired glucose tolerance of pregnancy in Riyadh. *British journal of obstetrics and gynaecology*, 95: 84–90.

Ahlquist DA et al. (1993) Accuracy of fecal occult blood screening for colorectal neoplasia: a prospective study using Hemoccult and HemoQuant tests. *Journal of the American Medical Association*, 269: 1262–1267.

Aluoch JA et al. (1984) Study of case-finding for pulmonary tuberculosis in outpatients complaining of chronic cough at a district hospital in Kenya. *American review of respiratory diseases*, 129: 915–920.

Anon. (1993) Drugs for AIDS and associated infections. *The medical letter*, 35(904): 79–86.

Arevalo JA, Washington AE (1988) Cost-effectiveness of prenatal screening and immunization for hepatitis B virus. *Journal of the American Medical Association*, 259(3): 365–369.

Ayangade O, Akinyemi A (1989) Cervical cytology in an urban Nigerian population. *East African medical journal*, 66(1): 50–56.

Aytekin AH, Saylan T (1988) Close-contact surveys and mass-screening studies for leprosy in Turkey. *Leprosy review*, 59: 225–229.

Backett EM et al. (1984) *The risk approach in health care.* Geneva, World Health Organization (Public Health Papers, No. 76).

Badami PV, Deodhar LP (1976) Asymptomatic bacteriuria in school children. *Journal of postgraduate medicine*, 22(3): 130–134.

Bain J (1990) Child health surveillance. *British medical journal*, 300: 1381–1382.

Barnes HV, ed. (1975) Symposium on adolescent medicine. *Medical clinics of North America*, 59: 4.

Battista RN, Lawrence RS, eds. (1988) *Implementing preventive services.* New York, Oxford University Press (supplement to *American journal of preventive medicine*).

Battista RN et al. (1984) The periodic health examination: 3. An evolving concept. *Canadian Medical Association journal*, 130:1288–1292.

Battista RN et al. (1991) The periodic health examination in the workplace. *Canadian family physician*, 37: 325–480.

Beers MH et al. (1991) Screening recommendations for the elderly. *American journal of public health*, 81(9): 1131–1140.

Bhat GJ et al. (1982) Congenital syphilis in Lusaka — III. Incidence in the neonatal intensive care unit. *East African medical journal*, 59(6): 374–378.

Braveman P, Toomey K (1987) Screening in preventive care for adolescents. *Western journal of medicine*, 146: 490–493.

Braveman P et al. (1988) Evaluating outcomes of pregnancy in diabetic women — epidemiologic considerations and recommended indicators. *Diabetes care*, 11: 281–287.

Brawer MK et al. (1992) Screening for prostate carcinoma with prostate-specific antigen. *Journal of urology*, 147: 841–845.

Britton WJ et al. (1987) The serological response to the phenolic glycolipid of *Mycobacterium leprae* in Australian and Nepali leprosy patients. *Australian and New Zealand journal of medicine*, 17(6): 568–573.

Browner W et al. (1991) What if Americans ate less fat? A quantitative estimate of the effect on mortality. *Journal of the American Medical Association*, 265(24): 3285–3291.

Bryers F, Hawthorne VM (1978) Screening for mild hypertension: costs and benefits. *Journal of epidemiology and community health*, 32(3): 171–174.

Burenkov SP, Glasunov IS (1982) USSR: the preventive approach in public health. *World health forum*, 3(1): 54–57.

Butler JR (1989) *Child health surveillance in primary care*. London, Crown.

CTF (1979) Canadian Task Force on the Periodic Health Examination. The periodic health examination. *Canadian Medical Association journal*, 121: 1193–1254.

CTF (1984) Canadian Task Force on the Periodic Health Examination. The periodic health examination: 2. 1984 update. *Canadian Medical Association journal*, 130: 1278–1285.

CTF (1986) Canadian Task Force on the Periodic Health Examination. The periodic health examination. 1985 update. *Canadian Medical Association journal*, 134: 724–729.

CTF (1989) Canadian Task Force on the Periodic Health Examination. The periodic health examination, 1989 update. *Canadian Medical Association journal*, Suppl.: 1–24.

CTF (1990) Canadian Task Force on the Periodic Health Examination. The periodic health examination, 1990 update. *Canadian Medical Association journal*, Suppl.: 1–23.

CTF (1991) Canadian Task Force on the Periodic Health Examination. The periodic health examination, 1991 update. *Canadian Medical Association journal*, Suppl.

Chamberlain J (1971) Multiple screening. *Community health*, 3(1): 17–23.

Chamberlain JM (1984) Which prescriptive screening programmes are worth while? *Journal of epidemiology and community health*, 38: 270–277.

CLAP (Centro LatinoAmericano de Perinatologia) (1987) Historia del sistema informatica perinatal. Montevideo, Uruguay, 1987. *Boletin del Centro LatinoAmericano de Perinatologia y Desarrollo Humano (CLAP) de OPS/OMS*, 2(8): 81–87.

Collaborative Study Group of Child Developmental Test (1986) Restandardization of DDST from six cities in north China. *Chinese medical journal*, 99: 166–172.

Cooper B, Bickel H (1984) Population screening and the early detection of dementing disorders in old age: a review. *Psychological medicine*, 14(1): 81–95.

Cooppan RM et al. (1987) Urinalysis reagent strips in the screening of children for urinary schistosomiasis in the RSA. *South African medical journal*, 72: 459–462.

Corth SB, Harris RW (1984) Incidence of middle ear disease in Indochinese refugee schoolchildren. *Audiology*, 23: 27–37.

Creese A, Parker D, eds. (1994) *Cost analysis in primary health care: a training manual for programme managers*. Geneva, World Health Organization.

Dawson P et al. (1976) Cost-effectiveness of screening children in housing projects. *American journal of public health*, 66: 1192–1194.

Dearlove J, Kearney D (1990) How good is general practice developmental screening? *British medical journal*, 300: 1177–1180.

Desai MP et al. (1987) Neonatal screening for congenital hypothyroidism in a developing country: problems and strategies. *Indian journal of pediatrics*, 54: 571–581.

D'Souza P et al. (1987) Primary school teachers in delivery of eye health care. *Indian journal of ophthalmology*, 35: 429–430.

Eddy DM et al. (1983) The value of screening for glaucoma with tonometry. *Survey of ophthalmology*, 28: 194–205.

Elegbe IA et al. (1987) Screening for urinary tract infections in asymptomatic elementary school children in Ile-Ife, Nigeria. *Journal of tropical pediatrics*, 33: 249–253.

Eliakim R et al. (1988) Screening for fecal occult blood in Israel. *Journal of clinical gastroenterology*, 10: 173–175.

Emery DD, Schneiderman LJ (1989) Cost-effectiveness analysis in health care. *Hastings Center Report*, July/August, 8–13.

Emmanuel JC et al. (1988) Pooling of sera for human immunodeficiency virus (HIV) testing: an economical method for use in developing countries. *Journal of clinical pathology*, 41: 582–585.

Engineer AD, Misra JS (1987) The role of routine outpatient cytological screening for early detection of carcinoma of the cervix in India. *Diagnostic cytopathology*, 3(1): 30–34.

Fernandez L et al. (1986) Risk factors in mass screening for breast cancer, multivariate analysis of data from the Cuban diagnosis pilot study. *Neoplasma*, 33: 535–541.

Fillenbaum GG (1985) *The wellbeing of the elderly; approaches to multidimensional assessment*. Geneva, World Health Organization (WHO Offset Publication No. 84).

Finau SA, Taylor L (1988) Rheumatic heart disease and school screening: initiatives at an isolated hospital in Tonga. *Medical journal of Australia*, 148: 563–567.

Flancbaum L et al. (1978) "Sidewalk" blood-pressure screening. effective and low-cost method. *New York State journal of medicine*, 78(6): 944–948.

Frame PS, Carlson SJ (1975) A critical review of periodic health screening using specific criteria. Parts 1–4. *Journal of family practice*, 1:29–36, 123–129, 189–194, 283–289.

Frank JW, Mai V (1985) Breast self-examination in young women: more harm than good? *Lancet*, 2(8456): 654–657.

Freer CB (1990) Screening the elderly. *British medical journal*, 300: 1447–1448.

Friedman Z et al. (1983) Ophthalmic screening of 38,000 children, age 1 to $2\frac{1}{2}$ years in child welfare clinics. *Journal of pediatric ophthalmology and strabismus*, 17(4): 261–267.

Ganapati R et al. (1984) Leprosy detection through non-survey techniques. *Indian journal of leprosy*, 45(3): 622–625.

Garud MA et al. (1983) Cytology screening program in an urban and rural community in India: review of a ten-year experience. *Acta cytologica*, 27(4): 429–431.

Gatner EMS, Burkhardt KR (1980) Correlation of the results of X-ray and sputum culture in tuberculosis prevalence surveys. *Tubercle*, 61: 27–31.

Goldbloom R, Battista RN (1986) The periodic health examination: 1. Introduction. *Canadian Medical Association journal*, 134: 721–723.

Gottlieb LK et al. (1983) Glaucoma screening. A cost-effectiveness analysis. *Survey of ophthalmology*, 28: 206–226.

Gottridge J et al. (1989) The nonutility of chest roentgenographic examination in asymptomatic patients with positive tuberculin test results. *Archives of internal medicine*, 149: 1660–1662.

Grace HJ (1981) Prenatal screening for neural tube defects in South Africa. *South African medical journal*, 60: 324–329.

Griffiths KD et al. (1982) Neonatal screening for sickle haemoglobinopathies in Birmingham. *British medical journal*, 284: 933–935.

Gunderson M et al. (1989) *AIDS: testing and privacy*. Salt Lake City, University of Utah Press.

Habbema JDF (1990) Screening for cervical and breast cancer in the Netherlands: policy and technology assessment. In: Jönsson B et al., eds. *Policy-making in health care. Changing goals and new tools*. Linköping, Linköping University, Faculty of Health Sciences (Health Service Studies 4).

Halberstam MJ (1970) The silent debits of multiphasic screening. *New England journal of medicine*, 283(20): 1114.

Hall DMB (1989) *Health for all children: a programme for child health surveillance*. Oxford, Oxford University Press.

Hamburg BA (1989) Adolescent health care and disease prevention in the Americas. In: Hamburg D, Sartorius N, eds. *Health and behaviour: selected perspectives*. Cambridge, Cambridge University Press :127–149.

Hart RH et al. (1990) *Integrating maternal and child health services with primary health care. Practical considerations*. Geneva, World Health Organization.

Hathaway WE et al., eds. (1991) *Current pediatric diagnosis and treatment*. East Norwalk, CT, Appleton & Lange.

Henderson JB (1982) Measuring the benefits of screening for open neural tube defects. *Journal of epidemiology and community health*, 36: 214–219.

Hoeper EW et al. (1984) The usefulness of screening for mental illness. *Lancet*, 1: 33–35.

Holland WW, Stewart S (1990) *Screening in health care*. London, Nuffield Provincial Hospitals Trust.

Holtzman NA (1991) What drives neonatal screening programs? *New England journal of medicine*, 325(11): 802–804.

Huang SC et al. (1988) Effectiveness of scoliometer in school screening for scoliosis. *Journal of the Formosan Medical Association*, 87: 955–959.

Imperato PJ et al. (1973) Mass campaigns and their comparative costs for nomadic and sedentary populations in Mali. *Tropical and geographical medicine*, 25: 416–422.

Institute of Medicine (1985) *Preventing low birthweight*. Washington, DC, National Academy Press.

Institute of Medicine (1988) *Prenatal care. Reaching mothers, reaching infants*. Washington, DC, National Academy Press.

Jenkins S (1990) Organisation of screening: a practical view. *British medical journal*, 300: 1050–1052.

Kan Guanqing (1981) Tuberculosis and its control in Beijing. *Chinese medical journal*, 94(10): 685–690.

Kasongo Project Team (1984) Antenatal screening for fetopelvic dystocias. A cost-effectiveness approach to the choice of simple indicators for use by auxiliary personnel. *Journal of tropical medicine and hygiene*, 87: 173–183.

Khare CB et al. (1988) Vignette method for psychiatric case detection in a rural community. *Medical journal of Malaysia*, 43: 100–107.

Kolata G (1985) Debate over colon cancer screening. *Science*, 229: 636–637.

Koroltchouk V et al. (1990) The control of breast cancer: a World Health Organization perspective. *Cancer*, 65(12): 2803–2810.

Krishnamoorthy K et al. (1985) Mass blood survey in three villages of Rameswaram Island endemic for malaria. *India journal of medical research*, 81: 140–142.

Krivinka R et al. (1974) Epidemiological and clinical study of tuberculosis in the district of Kolin, Czechoslovakia. *Bulletin of the World Health Organization*, 51: 59–69.

Laszlo J (1974) Automated "chemistries", a multiphasic misadventure (editorial). *Archives of internal medicine*, 133: 1068–1069.

Lengeler C et al. (1991a) Community-based questionnaires and health statistics as tools for the cost-efficient identification of communities at risk of urinary schistosomiasis (198) *International journal of epidemiology*, 20(3): 796–807.

Lengeler C et al. (1991b) Rapid, low-cost, two-step method to screen for urinary schistosomiasis at the district level: the Kilosa experience. *Bulletin of the World Health Organization*, 69(2): 179–189.

Levin B (1992) Screening sigmoidoscopy for colorectal cancer. *New England journal of medicine*, 326(6): 700–702.

Li HP et al. (1985) Early diagnosis of scoliosis based on school screening. *Journal of bone and joint surgery*, 8(67-A): 1202–1205.

Lima BR et al. (1987) Screening for the psychological consequences of a major disaster in a developing country: Armero, Colombia. *Acta psychiatrica scandinavica*, 76: 561–567.

Liu SR, Zuo QH (1986) Newborn screening for phenylketonuria in eleven districts. *Chinese medical journal*, 99: 113–118.

Louria DB et al. (1976) Primary and secondary prevention among adults: an analysis with comments on screening and health education. *Preventive medicine*, 5: 549–572.

Lozoff B et al. (1991) Long-term developmental outcome of infants with iron deficiency. *New England journal of medicine*, 325: 687–694.

Luka-Tombekana M (1984) *The role of medical auxiliaries in operative obstetrics in rural Zaire.* London, Institute of Child Health (dissertation).

Lunt R (1984) Worldwide early detection of cervical cancer. *Obstetrics and gynecology*, 63: 708–713.

Luthra UK et al. (1988) Clinical downstaging of uterine cervix by paramedical personnel. *Lancet*, 1: 1402.

Lynch HT et al. (1985) A demonstration project on cancer screening in rural Thailand: preliminary report. *Oncology*, 42: 193–197.

Macfarlane A et al. (1989) *Child health. The screening tests.* Oxford, Oxford University Press.

Manderson L, Aaby P (1992) Can rapid anthropological procedures be applied to tropical diseases? *Health policy and planning*, 7(1): 46–55.

Mathai M (1988) Prediction of small-for-gestational-age infants using a specially calibrated tape measure. *British journal of obstetrics and gynaecology*, 95: 313–314.

McCreary CH (1968) Tuberculosis control in India. *Diseases of the chest*, 53(6): 699–708.

McKeown T, Lowe CR, eds. (1974) *An introduction to social medicine*, 2nd ed. Oxford, Blackwell Scientific.

McNeil B et al. (1981) A cost-effectiveness analysis of screening for hepatitis B surface antigen in India. *Medical decision-making*, 1(4): 345–359.

McPherson BD, Holborow CA (1988) School screening for hearing loss in developing countries. *Scandinavian audiology*, 28(Suppl.): 103–110.

Miller AB (1989) Mammography: a critical evaluation of its role in breast cancer screening, especially in developing countries. *Journal of public health policy*, 487–497.

Miller AB (1991) The role of screening in the fight aganist breast cancer. *World health forum*, 13: 277–285.

Miller AB (1992) *Cervical cancer screening programmes: managerial guidelines*. Geneva, World Health Organization.

Modell B et al. (1991) *Community genetics services in Europe*. Copenhagen, WHO Regional Office for Europe.

Morrison B (1986) The periodic health examination: 3. Breast cancer. *Canadian Medical Association journal*, 134: 727–729.

Mott KE et al. (1985) Indirect screening for *Schistosoma haematobium* infection: a comparative study in Ghana and Zambia. *Bulletin of the World Health Organization*, 63(1): 135–142.

Mountin JW (1950) Multiple screening and specialized programs. *Public health reports*, 65(42): 1359–1368.

Mustafi AA, Kouris K (1985) Effective dose equivalent and associated risks from mass chest radiography in Kuwait. *Health physics*, 49(6): 1147–1154.

Nabarro D, Chinnock P (1988) Growth monitoring — inappropriate promotion of an appropriate technology. *Social science and medicine*, 26(9): 941–948.

Newman T et al. (1990) The case against childhood cholesterol screening. *Journal of the American Medical Association*, 264(23): 3039–3043.

Ng CSA et al. (1981) Diabetic screening in pregnancy. *Singapore medical journal*, 22(2): 59–63.

Nuffield Provincial Hospitals Trust (1968) *Screening in medical care. Reviewing the evidence*. London, Oxford University Press.

Oduwole OO, Ogunyemi AO (1989) Validity of the GHQ-30 in a Nigerian medical outpatient clinic. *Canadian journal of psychiatry*, 34: 20–23.

Ohwovoriole AE et al. (1988) Casual blood glucose levels and prevalence of undiscovered diabetes mellitus in Lagos Metropolis Nigerians. *Diabetes research and clinical practice*, 4: 153–158.

Okunade AO (1980) Screening for handicaps in children; are Nigerian nurses equipped? *International journal of nursing studies*, 17: 181–187.

Oviasu VO, Okupa FE (1980) Arterial blood pressure and hypertension in Benin in the equatorial forest zone of Nigeria. *Tropical and geographical medicine*, 32(3): 241–244.

PAHO (1984) *Prevention and control of genetic diseases and congenital defects*. Washington, DC, Pan American Health Organization (Scientific Publication, No. 460).

PAHO (1986) *Tuberculosis control: a manual on methods and procedures for integrated programs*. Washington, DC, Pan American Health Organization (Scientific Publication, No. 498).

Pandav CS, Kochupillai N (1985) Organisation and implementation of neonatal hypothyroid screening programme in India — a primary health care approach. *Indian journal of pediatrics*, 52: 223–229.

Pavlov KA, Semiglazov VF (1981) Detection of early forms of breast cancer by mass screening examinations. *Neoplasma*, 28: 611–615.

Paxman JM, Zuckerman RJL (1987) *Laws and policies affecting adolescent health*. Geneva, World Health Organization.

Peresra HW (1978) Choice of a policy in case finding. *Journal of the Nepal Medical Association*, 16(1): 72–82.

Pernoll ML, ed. (1991) *Current obstetric and gynecologic diagnosis and treatment*. East Norwalk, CT, Appleton & Lange.

Persaud V (1987) Screening for breast cancer saves lives. *West Indian medical journal*, 36: 57–59.

Phaff JML, ed. (1986) *Perinatal health services in Europe: searching for better childbirth*. London, Croom Helm.

Pierce C (1992) Jury still out on carotid endarterectomy. *Family practice news*, 22(20): 39–41.

Pinotti JA et al. (1981) Preventive obstetric and gynecology program: pilot plan for integrated medical care. *Bulletin of the Pan American Health Organization*, 15(2): 104–112.

Polnay L (1989) Child health surveillance — new report highlights value of parental observations. *British medical journal*, 299: 1351–1352.

Pratinidhi AK et al. (1987) Screening tests for vitamin A deficiency. *Indian journal of pediatrics*, 54: 563–570.

Program for Appropriate Technology in Health (1984a) Technologies for pregnancy care. *Health technology directions*, 4(1): 1–12.

Program for Appropriate Technology in Health (1984b) Technologies for safe birth. *Health technology directions*, 4(2): 1–16.

Program for Appropriate Technology in Health (1987) Iodine deficiency disorders. *Health technology directions*, 7(1):5.

Rai SK et al. (1987) Difference in tuberculin reaction read after forty-eight and seventy-two hours: a preliminary study. *Nepal Paediatrics Society journal*, 6(2): 13–15.

Roemer MI (1984) The value of medical care for health promotion. *American journal of public health*, 74(3): 243–248.

Royston E, Armstrong S, eds. (1989) *Preventing maternal deaths*. Geneva, World Health Organization.

Sampaio Goes J et al. (1981) Cervical cancer prevention and control in developing countries: a model program. *Bulletin of the Pan American Health Organization*, 15(3): 216–225.

Sarda RK et al. (1986) Further observations on the use of gross haematuria as an indirect screening technique for the detection of *Schistosoma haematobium* infection in school children in Dar es Salaam, Tanzania. *Journal of tropical medicine and hygiene*, 89: 309–312.

Sarue PHE et al. (1984) *El concepto de riesgo y el cuidado de la salud. Manual basico de aprendizaje inicial*. Montevideo, CLAP, American Institute of the Child.

Scheffler RM, Paringer L (1980) A review of the economic evidence on prevention. *Medical care*, XVIII(5): 473–484.

Schneider A, Meinhardt G (1984) Screening for cervical cancer in Butha Buthe, Lesotho. *Tropical doctor*, 14: 170–174.

Schroeder SA et al., eds. (1991) *Current medical diagnosis and treatment*. East Norwalk, CT, Appleton & Lange.

Selby JV et al. (1992) A case-control study of screening sigmoidoscopy and mortality from colorectal cancer. *New England journal of medicine*, 326: 653–657.

Semiglazov VF, Moissenko VM (1987) Breast self-examination for the early detection of breast cancer: a USSR/WHO controlled trial in Leningrad. *Bulletin of the World Health Organization*, 65(3): 391–396.

Sen B et al. (1987) Psychiatric morbidity in primary health care. A 2-stage screening procedure in developing countries. *British journal of psychiatry*, 151: 33–38.

Shah KP, Shah PM (1981) The mother's card: a simplified aid for primary health workers. *WHO chronicle*, 35(2): 51–53.

Shah PM et al. (1988) The home-based maternal record - a tool for family involvement in health care. *IPPF medical bulletin*, 22: 2–3.

Shrestha SM (1987) Incidence of HBsAg carrier rate in pregnant women in Kathmandu. *Journal of the institute of medicine*, 9: 71–76.

Shrivastav P et al. (1986) Selective screening for carcinoma cervix in South Indian women. *International journal of gynaecology and obstetrics*, 24(5): 337–342.

Silverberg DS et al. (1974) Use of shopping centres in screening for hypertension. *Canadian Medical Association journal*, 111: 769–774.

Singer B, Sawyer DO (1992) Perceived malaria illness reports in mobile populations. *Health policy and planning*, 7(1): 40–45.

Slater PE et al. (1981) The early breast cancer detection program of the Israel cancer association: a retrospective evaluation. *Israel journal of medical sciences*, 17: 827–838.

Smith GS (1989) Development of rapid epidemiologic assessment methods to evaluate health status and delivery of health services. *International journal of epidemiology*, 18(Suppl. 2): S2-S15.

Soni S, Ingle P (1982) Comparison of slum survey, school survey and health education as methods of detection of leprosy cases in urban area. *Leprosy in India*, 54(4): 716–720.

Spitzer WO (1984) The periodic health examination: 1. Introduction. *Canadian Medical Association journal*, 130: 1276–1278.

Stanley K, Stjernswärd J (1986) A survey on the control of oral cancer in India. *Indian journal of cancer*, 23: 105–111.

Stanley K et al. (1987) Women and cancer. *World health statistics quarterly*, 40: 267–278.

Sterky G et al., eds. (1985) *Breathing and warmth at birth: judging the appropriateness of technology.* Stockholm, Swedish Agency for Research Cooperation with Developing Countries.

Stewart TH (1966) Are mass miniature X-ray surveys among South African whites warranted? *South African medical journal*, 49(21): 493–495.

Stilma JS et al. (1983) Eye screening in 2234 Sierra Leonean school students and detection of onchocerciasis. *Documenta ophthalmologica*, 56: 123–129.

Stjernswärd J et al. (1987) Plotting a new course for cervical cancer screening in developing countries. *World health forum*, 8: 42–45.

Stray-Pedersen B (1983) Economic evaluation of maternal screening to prevent congenital syphilis. *Sexually transmitted diseases*, October-December.

Sun T-T et al. (1986) A pilot study on universal immunization of newborn infants in an area of hepatitis B virus and primary hepatocellular carcinoma prevalence with a low dose of hepatitis B vaccine. *Journal of cellular and comparative physiology*, 4: 83–90.

Taiwan Department of Health (1988) The Executive Yuan. The Taiwan program to strengthen the vision health care for the school children. *Acta ophthalmologica*, 185(Suppl.): 148–150.

Tanner M et al. (1987) Longitudinal study on the health status of children in a rural Tanzanian community: parasitoses and nutrition following control measures against intestinal parasites. *Acta tropica*, 44: 137–174.

Tao S et al. (1984) Twenty-three years' research on prevention of cervical cancer. *Chinese medical journal*, 97(5): 379–384.

Tarimo E, Fowkes FGR (1989) Strengthening the backbone of primary health care. *World health forum*, 10: 74–79.

Tatara K et al. (1991) Relation between use of health check ups starting in middle age and demand for inpatient care by elderly people in Japan. *British medical journal*, 302: 615–618.

Teklu B, Kassegn K (1982) Mass miniature radiography at the tuberculosis demonstration and training centre, Addis Ababa. *Ethiopian medical journal*, 20: 131–134.

Terris M (1981) The primacy of prevention. *Preventive medicine*, 10: 689–699.

Thompson MS et al. (1981) Cost-effectiveness of screening for hypo- and hyperthyroidism in India. *Medical decision-making*, 1(1): 44–58.

Trachtenberg AI et al. (1988) A cost-based decision analysis for chlamydia screening in California family planning clinics. *Obstetrics and gynecology*, 71: 101–108.

Trowbridge FL, Staehling N (1980) Sensitivity and specificity of arm circumference indicators in identifying malnourished children. *American journal of clinical nutrition*, 33: 687–696.

Tsega E et al. (1987) Prevalence of hepatitis B virus markers among Ethiopian blood donors: is HBsAg screening necessary? *Tropical and geographical medicine*, 39: 336–340.

Tuke JW (1990) Screening and surveillance of school aged children. *British medical journal*, 300: 1180–1182.

Tuomilehto J et al. (1987) Sequels to screening for HTN and MM in Fiji. *Diabetes research and clinical practice*, 4: 15–22.

United Nations (1986) *How to weigh and measure children. Assessing the nutritional status of young children in household surveys.* New York (Annex 1: Summary procedures).

USPSTF (1989) United States Preventive Services Task Force. *Guide to clinical preventive services*. Baltimore, MD, Williams and Wilkins.

USDHEW (1971) National Center for Health Services Research and Development. *Multiphasic health testing systems: reviews and annotations.* Rockville, MD, US Government Printing Office (HSRD 71-1).

van der Maas PJ et al. (1989) The cost-effectiveness of breast cancer screening. *International journal of cancer*, 43: 1055–1060.

Venkataswamy G (1972) Eye camps in India. *Israel journal of medical sciences*, 8(8-9): 1254–1259.

Vlassoff C, Tanner M (1992) The relevance of rapid assessment to health research and interventions. *Health policy and planning*, 7(1): 1–9.

Wang YY, Yang S (1985) Occult impaired hearing among 'normal' school children in endemic goiter and cretinism areas due to iodine deficiency in Guizhou. *Chinese medical journal*, 98(2): 89–94.

Warnakulasuriya KAAS et al. (1983) Can primary health workers screen for oral cancer? *World health forum*, 4(3): 202–204.

Warnakulasuriya KAAS et al. (1984) Utilization of primary health care workers for early detection of oral cancer and precancer cases in Sri Lanka. *Bulletin of the World Health Organization*, 62(2): 243–250.

Warnakulasuriya S et al. (1988) Compliance following referral in the early detection of oral cancer and precancer in Sri Lanka. *Community dentistry and oral epidemiology*, 16(6): 326–329.

Watson-Williams EJ et al. (1988) Solid phase red cell adherence immunoassay for anti-HIV-1: a simple, rapid, and accurate method for donor screening. *Transfusion*, 28(2): 184–186.

Way LW, ed. (1988) *Current surgical diagnosis and treatment*. East Norwalk, CT, Appleton and Lange.

WHO (1971) *Report of the Technical Discussions at the Twenty-fourth World Health Assembly on "Mass Health Examinations as a Public Health Tool"*. Geneva, World Health Organization (A24 Tech. Discussions).

WHO (1975) *Early detection of health impairment in occupational exposure to health hazards: report of a WHO Study Group*. Geneva, World Health Organization (WHO Technical Report Series, No. 571).

WHO (1976) *Epidemiology of onchocerciasis: report of a WHO Expert Committee*. Geneva, World Health Organization (WHO Technical Report Series, No. 597).

WHO (1983) *Prevention of liver cancer: report of a WHO Meeting*. Geneva, World Health Organization (WHO Technical Report Series, No. 691)

WHO (1984a) *Task force on appropriate technology for pregnancy and perinatal care. Report of the first meeting of the steering committee*. Geneva, World Health Organization (unpublished document WHO/FHE/MCH 84.2 Rev.1; available on request from Maternal and Child Health, World Health Organization, 1211 Geneva 27, Switzerland).

WHO (1984b) *Strategies for the prevention of blindness in national programmes. A primary health care approach*. Geneva, World Health Organization.

WHO (1985a) *Having a baby in Europe*. Copenhagen, WHO Regional Office for Europe.

WHO (1986a) *Early detection of occupational diseases*. Geneva, World Helath Organization.

WHO (1986b) *Scales and related techniques for weighing pregnant women, newborns, infants and children: an evaluation*. Geneva, World Health Organization (unpublished document WHO/FHE/MCH 86.5; available on request from Maternal and Child Health, World Health Organization, 1211 Geneva 27, Switzerland).

WHO (1986c) *The growth chart. A tool for use in infant and child health care*. Geneva, World Health Organization.

WHO (1987) *Birth weight surrogates. The relationship between birth weight, arm and chest circumference*. Geneva, World Health Organization (unpublished document WHO/FHE/MCH 87.8; available on request from Maternal and Child Health, World Health Organization, 1211 Geneva 27, Switzerland).

WHO (1988) *The challenge of implementation: district health systems for primary health care*. Geneva, World Health Organization (WHO/SHS/DHS/88.1/Rev. 1; available on request from Strengthening of Health Services, World Health Organization, 1211 Geneva 27, Switzerland).

WHO (1989a) *Report on workshop on home-based mother's records, February 1989.* Manila, WHO Regional Office for Western Pacific (document WHO ROWP 1989)

WHO (1989b) *Health of the elderly: report of a WHO Expert Committee.* Geneva, World Health Organization (WHO Technical Report Series, No. 779).

WHO (1989c) *Interim evaluation of the USSR/WHO study of breast self-examination in breast cancer early detection.* Geneva, World Health Organization. (unpublished document WHO/CAN/ BSE/89; available on request from Cancer, World Health Organization, 1211 Geneva 27, Switzerland).

WHO (1993a) *A global strategy for malaria control.* Geneva, World Health Organization.

WHO (1993b) *Implementation of the global malaria control strategy: report of a WHO Study Group.* Geneva, World Health Organization (WHO Technical Report Series, No. 839).

WHO (1994) *Home-based maternal records. Guidelines for development, adaptation and evaluation.* Geneva, World Health Organization.

WHO Meeting (1984) Control of oral cancer in developing countries. *Bulletin of the World Health Organization,* 62: 817–830.

WHO Meeting (1986) Control of cancer of the cervix uteri. *Bulletin of the World Health Organization,* 64: 607–618.

WHO/UNICEF (1978) *Primary health care. Report of the International Conference on Primary Health Care, Alma-Ata, 1978.* Geneva, World Health Organization ("Health for All" Series, No. 1).

WHO/UNICEF (1986) *Maternal care for the reduction of perinatal and neonatal mortality. A joint WHO/UNICEF statement.* Geneva, World Health Organization.

Wilson JMG (1971) *Background document based on summary reports received from countries and other material for reference and use at the Technical Discussions on "Mass Health Examinations as a Public Health Tool".* Geneva, World Health Organization (unpublished document A24/Technical Discussions/1)

Wilson JMG, Jungner G (1968) *Principles and practice of screening for disease.* Geneva, World Health Organization (Public Health Papers, No. 34).

Winawer SJ, Miller D (1987) Screening for colorectal cancer. *Bulletin of the World Health Organization,* 65: 105–110.

Wu Y et al. (1981) A five year report on community control of hypertension, stroke and coronary heart disease in the Shijingshan people's commune, Beijing. *Chinese medical journal,* 94(4): 233–236.

Wu Y et al. (1982) Nation-wide hypertension screening in China during 1979-1980. *Chinese medical journal,* 95(2): 101–108.

Yang D et al. (1985) Mass cytologic screening for cervical carcinoma in China. *Acta cytologica,* 29(3): 341–344.

Yelland A et al. (1991) Diagnosing breast carcinoma in young women. *British medical journal,* 302: 618–620

Zadik Z et al. (1987) Blood pressure determinations in Israeli schoolchildren aged 5 to 14 years. *Israel journal of medical sciences*, 23: 789–802.

Zhang G et al. (1988) Screening for scoliosis among school children in Beijing. *Chinese medical journal*, 101(2): 151–154.

Statement from the Consultation on Testing and Counselling for HIV Infection [1]

Geneva, 16–18 November 1992

I. Introduction

A reliable test for antibody to HIV (human immunodeficiency virus) was first developed in 1984 and became widely available in many parts of the world by 1985. The development of this test enabled researchers to understand HIV infection and AIDS better, allowed health care workers to diagnose HIV infection in patients, and gave individuals the choice of knowing whether or not they were infected with HIV. HIV infection, including AIDS, has important characteristics that affect the usefulness of HIV testing and distinguish it from testing for many other health conditions:

- HIV infection is lifelong, as is infectiousness, and there is at present no drug known to render infected individuals non-infectious. Therefore, unlike diseases such as syphilis, early diagnosis does not lead to any medical treatment to prevent transmission.
- HIV infection is believed to be eventually fatal in virtually all cases, with no known cure, although early therapy, if available, may delay the onset of various HIV-related diseases, and prolong life.
- HIV infection is not transmissible by casual contact. Nevertheless, because of ignorance of this fact, and because HIV is a fatal disease spread mainly through sexual intercourse, individuals known to be HIV-infected are often stigmatized and discriminated against.
- Because HIV is transmitted through modifiable behaviours, providing individuals with their test results on a voluntary basis and with appropriate counselling can, in some cases, promote behaviour change that is beneficial to the individual, as well as to public health.

These special characteristics of HIV infection have important implications for the potential role of HIV testing in HIV/AIDS prevention and care programmes.

In order to identify issues that should be considered in planning and implementing an HIV testing programme, WHO organized a meeting in Geneva in May 1987 on "Criteria for HIV screening programmes", which made recommendations on the role of various types of HIV testing programmes for HIV/AIDS prevention and care. More specifically, the meeting

---

[1] Reproduced from unpublished WHO document WHO/GPA/INF/93.2.

participants voiced concerns about the situation at that time with respect to HIV testing programmes, noting that:

> [screening] efforts may be driven by unfounded concerns about casual transmission of HIV or a need to appear to be taking visible action against the HIV problem. The purposes of the [testing] programmes and the objectives to be achieved are not always cleary defined and the practical, economic, and social costs of implementing such programmes may not have been clearly examined.

The participants also noted that:

> readily available counselling and testing for HIV, provided on a voluntary basis, are more likely to result in behaviour changes that contribute to the public health goal of reducing spread of HIV than are mandatory [testing] initiatives,

and noted, in conclusion that:

> [testing] by itself does not result in behaviour changes that restrict transmission of HIV to others. ... For effective prevention, all persons who are potentially at risk of infection must be included in the programme to reduce or eliminate risk behaviour, regardless of whether they are infected and whether they have been tested.

Although these observations and conclusions remain valid, additional information and experience have been gained since 1987 and approaches to the prevention of HIV transmission and the provision of care to those affected by HIV/AIDS have changed. The availability and reliability of HIV antibody tests have improved, and the cost of these tests has decreased. In addition, the HIV/AIDS pandemic has expanded to affect far more people, in more parts of the world.

In order to offer national AIDS programmes up-to-date guidance on the role of HIV testing and counselling of asymptomatic people, a consultation was held at WHO headquarters on 16–18 November 1992. Its purpose was to review what is known about the advantages and disadvantages of HIV testing, and to develop recommendations on the role of testing and counselling in HIV/AIDS prevention and care programmes.

The consultation specifically focused on the role of testing and counselling for the early detection of infection in asymptomatic people. It did not aim to provide guidance on the other purposes for which HIV testing is done, namely:

- Ensuring transfusion and transplantation safety by screening blood for transfusion, semen and ova for donation, and organs and tissues for transplantation (see: *Global Blood Safety Initiative. Consensus Statement on Screening of Blood Donations for Infectious Agents Transmissible through Blood Transfusion.* WHO/LBS/91.1).
- Epidemiological surveillance (see: *Unlinked Anonymous Screening for the Public Health Surveillance of HIV Infections. Proposed International Guidelines.* WHO/GPA/SFI/89.3).

- Research (see: *International Guidelines for Ethical Review of Epidemiological Studies* (Council for International Organizations of Medical Sciences [CIOMS], Geneva, 1991).
- Diagnosis of symptomatic infection (see: *Guidelines for the Clinical Management of HIV infection in Adults*. WHO/GPA/IDS/HCS/91.6).

II. Mandatory testing and other testing without informed consent

HIV testing can be classified as being done with or without informed consent. Mandatory testing and other testing without informed consent has no place in an AIDS prevention and control programme. The Forty-fifth World Health Assembly noted that

> there is no public health rationale for any measures that limit the rights of the individual, notably measures establishing mandatory screening (resolution WHA 45.35, 14 May 1992).

There are no benefits either to the individual or for public health arising from testing without informed consent that cannot be achieved by less intrusive means, such as voluntary testing and counselling.

Public health experience demonstrates that programmes that do not respect the rights and dignity of individuals are not effective. It is essential, therefore, to promote the voluntary cooperation of individuals rather than impose coercive measures upon them.

Furthermore, testing programmes that do not require and secure an individual's informed consent can be damaging to efforts to prevent HIV transmission — and are therefore not in the interest of public health — for the following reasons:

- Because of the stigmatization and discrimination directed at HIV-infected people, individuals who believe they might be infected tend to go "underground" to escape mandatory testing. As a result, those at highest risk for HIV infection may not hear or heed education messages about AIDS prevention.
- Testing without informed consent damages the credibility of the health services and may discourage those needing services from obtaining them.
- In any testing programme, there will be people who falsely test negative — for example, because of laboratory error or because they are infected but have not yet developed detectable antibodies to HIV. Thus, mandatory testing can never identify all HIV-infected people.
- Mandatory testing can create a false sense of security especially among people who are outside its scope and who use it as an excuse for not following more effective measures for protecting themselves and others from infection. Examples are health care workers who do not follow universal precautions when all hospital patients are tested, and clients of sex workers who do not use condoms when they believe that all prostitutes are being tested.

- Mandatory testing programmes are expensive, and divert resources from effective prevention measures.

Despite strong evidence that mandatory testing is not in the interest of public health, a number of mandatory testing programmes and other programmes not involving informed consent are currently in place or have been proposed by governments or legislative bodies. Of special note are programmes in which testing without informed consent may be initiated by a health care worker. Two important examples of populations tested in this way are:

- *Women of reproductive age, including pregnant women*: Women who are, or who might become, pregnant have sometimes been subjected to testing without informed consent, including mandatory testing, for the purpose of preventing childbirth or breast-feeding among those who are HIV-positive. However, testing without informed consent, even if provided confidentially, offers no advantage over voluntary testing and counselling programmes designed to assist women in making decisions about childbearing and/or breast-feeding. Those women who want to know if they are infected before making such decisions generally would participate in voluntary testing and counselling programmes. Furthermore, not only is it unethical to pressure or force women to make reproductive or breast-feeding decisions for any reason, including their HIV infection status, but those women most likely to be HIV-infected may try to avoid mandatory testing, precisely in order to avoid pressure in such decision-making. Such avoidance may have the additional unwanted result of discouraging pregnant women from attending antenatal services.
- *Patients*: Ambulatory and hospitalized patients have been subjected to testing without informed consent, including mandatory testing, on the grounds that this is necessary in order to allow health care workers to take precautions to prevent themselves and other patients from becoming infected. However, there is no role for testing without informed consent in the prevention of HIV transmission in the health care setting. Rather, the application of universal precautions in infection control procedures is the best way to minimize HIV transmission in the health care setting. The concept of universal precautions means that *all* blood (and other potentially infectious body fluids) is assumed to be infectious and standard infection control procedures should therefore be applied for *all* patients, regardless of whether an HIV test is positive, negative, or not done at all (see: *Report of a WHO Consultation on the Prevention of Human Immunodeficiency Virus and Hepatitis B Virus Transmission in the Health Care Setting.* WHO/GPA/DIR/91.5). The testing of patients, in particular those with sexually transmitted disease, has also been advocated so that those who are infected can be offered appropriate counselling and other care. However, this purpose can be accomplished through *voluntary* testing and counselling (see Section III, below). The only other role of HIV testing for patients is to assist in making a diagnosis of HIV infection when this is suggested by clinical signs and symptoms. Testing without informed consent holds no advantage over testing with informed consent in such cases.

In many parts of the world, other populations have been, or are being, subjected to mandatory or other testing without consent. Again, although the rationale for mandatory testing — when stated — is often said to be related to health, in fact neither individual nor public health benefits result from such testing that cannot be better achieved through voluntary testing. Following is a non-exhaustive list of such groups:

- Population groups considered to be at high risk of HIV infection, such as injecting drug users, prostitutes, homosexual men, and prisoners (see: *WHO Guidelines on HIV Infection and AIDS in Prisons.* WHO/GPA/DIR/93.3)
- Military, including applicants and those already in service
- International travellers, including immigrants, refugees, returning emigrants (such as students), and guest workers (see: *Statement on Screening of International Travellers for Infection with Human Immunodeficiency Virus.* WHO/GPA/INF/88.3)
- People planning to marry
- Health care workers (see: *Report of a WHO Consultation on the Prevention of Human Immunodeficiency Virus and Hepatitis B Virus Transmission in the Health Care Setting,* cited above)
- Other workers (see: *Statement from the Consultation on AIDS and the Workplace.* WHO/GPA/INF/88.7)
- Athletes (see: *Consensus Statement from Consultation on AIDS and Sports.* WHO/GPA/INF/89.2)

Blood for transfusion should be screened for HIV. If screening is not anonymous and unlinked — i.e., if personal identifying data are kept with the specimen and the test results are to be made known to the donor — then the donor must be told this in advance and must give informed consent to such testing. Blood donation should not be mandatory nor carried out in such a way that people are pressured to donate, or are stigmatized if they self-defer (see: *Global Blood Safety Initiative. Consensus Statement on Screening of Blood Donations for Infectious Agents Transmissible through Blood Transfusion.* WHO/LBS/91.1).

The term "routine testing" is often used to refer to testing that is carried out unless the patient or client explicitly refuses — or is conducted without the subject even knowing. When routine testing carries either of these meanings, it represents an approach to testing that does not require pretest counselling and explicit consent. As a form of testing without informed consent, it is ineffective and unethical.

III. Voluntary testing and counselling

Voluntary testing accompanied by counselling has a place within a comprehensive range of measures for HIV/AIDS prevention, care and support. However, it must always be justified in terms of the balance of advantages and disadvantages to the individual who is tested. Within the context of a well-designed confidential counselling programme, voluntary testing may be of net benefit for those individuals who wish to know whether or not they are HIV-infected. However, it should be borne in mind that counselling on its own is a valuable intervention even if HIV testing is not available or if the client decides not to be tested. The potential benefits of counselling to the individual include:

- receiving accurate information about HIV
- becoming more able to cope with anxiety
- receiving emotional support
- learning methods of risk reduction
- becoming motivated and/or empowered to initiate risk-reduction behaviours
- having risk-reduction behaviours reinforced
- receiving referral to additional medical or social support services.

These benefits are likely to be enhanced where preventive measures (e.g., condom supply) and supportive measures (e.g., provision of food, shelter, home care) are available and where the social environment is favourable towards people affected by HIV.

Voluntary testing with counselling has the following potential advantages over and above counselling alone:

- having the knowledge of one's serostatus
- relieving anxiety associated with uncertainty
- if HIV-infected, being referred to clinical care and receiving specific drug therapy, where this is available
- planning for the future — e.g., for the care of children and the setting of one's affairs in order, and making decisions about childbearing, breast-feeding, and future relationships
- possibly enhanced motivation for risk reduction, and a more informed choice concerning personal preventive strategy.

Some individuals may *not* want to know whether or not they are HIV-infected, for various reasons — for example, because they believe that this knowledge would have little impact on their behavioural decisions, and/or might lead to greatly increased anxiety (especially if infected). Counselling should be provided for these individuals if they so desire.

The evidence that voluntary HIV testing may play a role in the prevention of transmission is not conclusive, except for discordant couples (i.e., where one partner is infected and the other uninfected), in whom it has been shown to result in less risky behaviour in those settings studied. Testing in itself is not a preventive measure; it could in principle aid prevention in other settings only if it succeeds in motivating individuals to adopt or maintain safer behaviours. Individuals are more likely to be thus motivated if they believe that HIV testing is of great benefit to themselves, such as when testing is provided in the context of a comprehensive counselling programme, with care and support services available, in a favourable social environment, and when the test is client-initiated.

Essential components of voluntary testing and counselling

To be beneficial, voluntary HIV testing, whether client- or health worker-initiated, must be:

1. *part of a comprehensive counselling programme*, in which trained counsellors provide counselling before a decision is made about testing (pre-test counselling), and provide counselling along with other supportive services (such as the provision of condoms and safer injecting equipment, where appropriate) or referral after testing (post-test counselling). The objectives of counselling should be:
   - to allow the expression of concerns and emotions about individual risks and behaviour
   - to clarity technical aspects of testing and assess the need for testing
   - to explore the implications of the test results for the individual, and to assess the individual's capacity to cope with such implications
   - to provide support, guidance, and referral, as needed.
2. *entirely the choice of the individual* whether or not to be tested; only the individual, assisted by information provided by a counsellor, can make a decision regarding the relative advantages and disadvantages of HIV testing for him or herself (i.e., informed consent). The person's individual circumstances, and the larger social context, will affect the balance of advantages and drawbacks of testing for that individual at a particular time. There must be no coercion or pressure to be tested — otherwise HIV testing may be counterproductive for the individual and/or society and cannot be considered to be truly voluntary.
3. *confidential or anonymous*: any potential or real breach of confidentiality greatly diminishes the value of HIV testing for an individual.
4. *technically sound* in terms of the laboratory tests used and the quality of the laboratory practices.

Planning issues for national AIDS programmes

Voluntary HIV testing and counselling is of benefit in the care and support of individuals. It may therefore have an important role in national AIDS programmes within the spectrum of HIV/AIDS care and support strategies. However, further research is needed to determine what role voluntary HIV testing and counselling could play as part of national AIDS prevention activities. This should be studied in a variety of population groups and compared with data on other preventive interventions to determine its relative cost-effectiveness.

The current availability of HIV/AIDS counselling, of voluntary HIV testing, and of HIV counselling combined with voluntary testing varies greatly around the world. Where voluntary HIV testing is not yet widely available, national AIDS programmes should proceed cautiously in introducing it in order to ensure that confidentiality or anonymity is guaranteed and that the service can be delivered in a manner most likely to result in benefits to the individual and the public health. In the process of developing a national policy on HIV voluntary testing and counselling, where such services are not already available, a trial programme should ideally be initiated and evaluated to determine the demand for client-initiated services, programme cost, potential sustainability, and efficacy in supporting the client and/or facilitating preventive behaviour.

In areas where voluntary testing and counselling, or counselling alone, is already available, the impact of the existing programme should be evaluated, in terms of both its planned or intended effects and any unforeseen benefits or harm.

There are additional issues which should be considered in the decision to implement or maintain a voluntary testing and counselling programme. One is the level of HIV knowledge in the local population: in general, testing will offer greater benefits in communities where levels of awareness and knowledge are already high. Another important consideration is the existence of safeguards against human rights abuses for those tested and those who learn that they are seropositive.

IV. Summary

- Testing without informed consent should not be done, regardless of its rationale, the population group tested, or the term used to designate the testing programme.
- Voluntary testing and counselling can be useful in the care and support of seropositive individuals, can provide reassurance and support to seronegative individuals, and can relieve anxiety in both groups.
- Several studies have indicated that voluntary testing and counselling may be effective in preventing HIV transmission among discordant couples when both members of the couple voluntarily participate in the testing and counselling. For other groups or situations, findings are inconsistent, and more research is needed.
- National AIDS programmes that decide to develop voluntary testing and counselling services where none now exist should proceed cautiously by initiating and evaluating a trial project. Where such services already exist, their impact should be evaluated.

Index

Index